60 Hikes Within 60 miles: TWIN CITIES

For Ross,
Congratulations on
your graduation from
Waterville High & best
of luck at Macalester!

Fondly,
Caroline
June 2007

Dedication

In memory of my Dad, who guided me down that first outdoor path so many years ago.

60 Hikes Within 60 Miles:

TWIN CITIES

Tom Watson

1st Edition

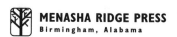

MENASHA RIDGE PRESS
Birmingham, Alabama

Library of Congress Cataloging-in-Publication Data

Watson, Tom, 1947–
    60 hikes within 60 miles: twin cities/Tom Watson.—1st ed.
        p. cm.
    1. Hiking—Minnesota—Minneapolis Metropolitan Area—Guidebooks.
    2. Hiking—Minnesota—Saint Paul Metropolitan Area—Guidebooks.
    3. Minneapolis Metropolitan Area (Minn.)—Guidebooks. I. Title: Sixty
    hikes within sixty miles. II. Title: Twin cities. III. Title.

ISBN 0-89732-411-0
ISBN 13 978-0-89732-411-3

GV199.42.M62 M569 2002
796.51'09776'579—dc21

                                                            2002024416

Cover and text design by Grant M. Tatum
Cover photo by Tom Watson
All interior photos by Tom Watson
Maps by Steve Jones and Bud Zehmer

Menasha Ridge Press
P.O. Box 43673
Birmingham, AL 35243
www.menasharidge.com

Table of Contents

vii
Map Legend
viii
Regional Map
x
Acknowledgments
xi
Foreword
xii
Preface
xv
Hiking Recommendations
xviii
Introduction
1
Afton State Park (# 1)
5
Ann Lake, Sand Dunes State Forest (#5)
8
Baker Park Reserve (#3)
12
Barn Bluff (# 4)
16
Bass Pond Trail, Long Meadow Lake (# 5)
20
Battle Creek (# 6)
23
Baylor Regional Park (# 7)
26
Bryant Lake Figure Eight (# 8)
29
City Lakes Chain, Lakes Harriet, Calhoun, and Isles (# 9)
33
Cleary Lake Regional Park (# 10)
37
Clifton E. French Regional Park (# 11)
40
Coon Rapids Dam (# 12)
43
Cottage Grove Ravine Regional Park (# 13)

47
Crosby Farm Park (# 14)
51
Crow-Hassen Regional Park (# 15)
55
Eastman Nature Trail (# 16)
60
Elm Creek Park Reserve (# 17)
64
Fish Lake Regional Park (# 18)
67
Fort Snelling State Park (Snelling Lake and Pine Island Trails) (# 19)
70
Frontenac State Park (Bluffside Trail) (# 20)
74
Hay Creek (West Trail) (# 21)
78
Hyland Lakes Park Reserve (Richardson Interpretive Trail) (# 22)
82
Interstate Park, Minnesota (# 23)
86
Interstate Park, Wisconsin (# 24)
91
Kinnickinnic State Park, Wisconsin (# 25)
94
Lake Byllesby Regional Park (# 26)
97
Lake Como, Como Park (# 27)
100
Lake Elmo Park Reserve, Eagle Point Lake (# 28)
103
Lake Maria State Park (# 29)
107
Lake Minnewashta Regional Park (Marsh Trail Loop) (# 30)
110
Lake Nokomis (# 31)

Table of Contents (continued)

114
Lake Phalen (# 32)

117
Lake Rebecca (# 33)

120
Lawrence Trail, Minnesota Valley (# 34)

124
Lebanon Hills Regional Park (Holland/
Jensen Lakes Loop) (# 35)

129
Long Lake (# 36)

133
Mazomani Trail, Louisville Swamp/
Minnesota Valley (# 37)

138
Miesville Ravine Park (# 38)

141
Minnehaha Falls and Creek (# 39)

145
Mississippi Gorge Trail (# 40)

149
Murphy-Hanrehan Park Reserve (# 41)

152
Nerstrand Big Woods State Park (Big
Woods Trail) (# 42)

156
Old Cedar Avenue Trail, Long Meadow
Lake (# 43)

160
Pine Point Park Trail (# 44)

163
Red Cedar Trail, Wisconsin (# 45)

167
Rice Creek Chain of Lakes Regional
Park Reserve (# 46)

170
Rice Lake State Park (# 47)

173
Rum River Central (# 48)

177
Rum River North (# 49)

180
Sakatah Lake State Park (# 50)

183
Sherburne NWR (Prairie's Edge Trail)
(# 51)

187
Snail Lake (# 52)

190
Spring Lake Park Reserve (Schaar's
Bluff Trail) (# 53)

194
Tamarack Nature Center (# 54)

197
Tamarack Trail, Lowry Nature Center/
Carver Park Reserve (# 55)

201
Thompson Trail, Thompson County
Park (# 56)

204
Wild River (# 57)

208
William O'Brien State Park (Upper
Park Trail) (# 58)

212
Willow River, Wisconsin (# 59)

216
Wood Lake Nature Center (# 60)

220
Appendix: Information Sources

222
Index

230
About the Author

MAP LEGEND

Main Trail

Alternate Trail

Interstate Highway

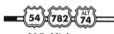
U.S. Highway

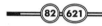
State Highway

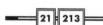
County Road

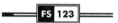
Forest Service Road

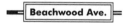
Local Road

Unpaved Road

Direction of Travel

Board Walk

State Border

County Border

Power Line

Park-Forest Boundary
and Label

Trailhead
Locator Map

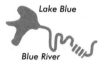
Water Features
Lake/Pond, Creek/River,
and Waterfall

Capitol, City, and Town

Peaks and Mountains

Footbridge/Dam,
Footbridge, and Dam

Tunnel

Swamp/Marsh

NORTH

35: Name of Hike

Map Scale
Compass, Map Number,
Name and Scale

Off Map or Pinpoint
Indication Arrow

Caution/Warning

Trailhead
for Specific Maps

Ranger Station/
Rest Room Facilities

Ranger Station

Rest Room Facilities

Shelter

Structure
or Feature

Monument/
Sculpture

Parking

Recreation Area

Metro Rail

Shuttle
Dropoff

Campgrounds

Picnic Area

Gate

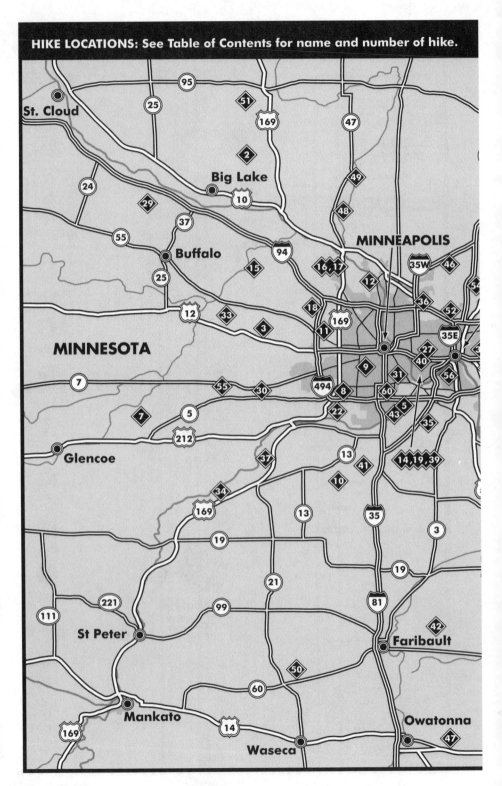

St. Cloud

95

25

51

169

47

2

Big Lake

49

24

29

48

10

MINNEAPOLIS

37

55

Buffalo

94

35W

46

15

16, 17

12

25

18

36

52

12

33

3

169

35E

MINNESOTA

11

27

40

35E

7

56

55

30

494

8

9

31

60

7

5

22

43

5

212

35

Glencoe

37

13

14, 19, 39

41

10

34

169

13

35

3

19

19

21

81

221

99

111

42

St Peter

Faribault

50

60

Mankato

169

14

47

Waseca

Owatonna

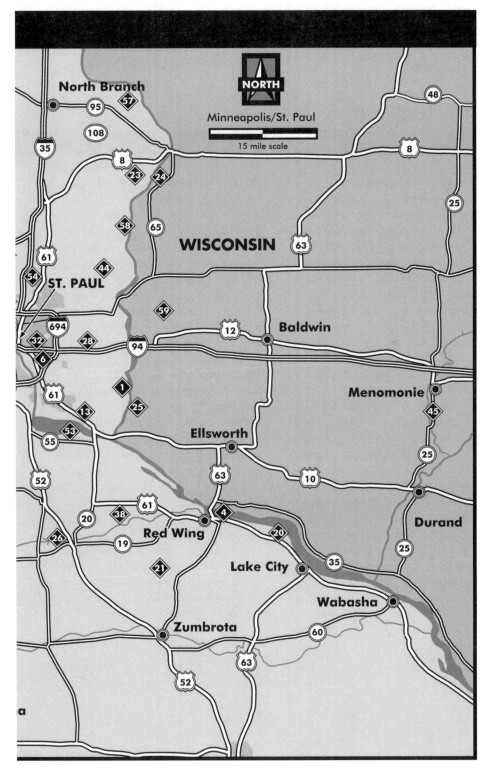

Acknowledgments

In this age of almost instantaneous information retrieval, I found all the agencies in the Twin Cities who manage trails within their respective boundaries are very well "wired" when it comes to providing up-to-date information. Websites and other contact numbers listed in the Appendix offer hikers a plethora of information on the trails and amenities of nearly every park in the Twin Cities.

Hennipen Parks, now known as Three Rivers Parks District, has an incredible resource base of maps and information about each park in their domain.

The Minnesota Valley National Wildlife Refuge offers a daisy-chain of park areas along the Minnesota River—one of the best scenic and wildlife viewing areas in the Twin Cities. Their information base, like their parks, continually improves, with more helpful maps and brochures each year.

More useful descriptions of hiking areas and amenities are provided by the U.S. Fish & Wildlife Service. I don't believe there is one federal agency responsible for outdoor recreation that doesn't have useful information on hiking opportunities in their management areas.

On a more localized basis, each county and municipality has published maps and information charts highlighting which parks offer hiking trails. Armed with this information and a good map of the cities, one can literally hike from one end to the other, guided all the way with neighborhood information on trails and amenities.

The tourism departments of both Minnesota and Wisconsin feature hiking as a predominant recreation activity in their respective states. Each offers maps and general information as well as contact information for each recreational region of their state.

Minnesota's Department of Natural Resources, particularly the great people at the state park system, is yet another incredible source of information. A good number of the hikes in this book are found within state parks close to the Twin Cities, and information provided by the DNR enables a hiker to get a feel for the entire state just by sampling trails at these nearby areas.

Very special thanks to my sister, Lynn, whose invaluable research, ongoing hospitality, and support throughout this project will always be deeply appreciated.

Foreword

Welcome to Menasha Ridge Press's *60 Hikes Within 60 Miles,* a series designed to provide hikers with the information they need to find and hike the very best trails surrounding cities usually under-served by guidebooks.

Our goal was simple: First, find a hiker who knows the area and loves to hike. Second, ask that person to spend a year researching the most popular and very best trails around. And third, have that person describe each trail in terms of difficulty, scenery, condition, elevation change, and other categories of information that are important to hikers. "Pretend you've just completed a hike and met up with other hikers at the trailhead," we told each author. "Imagine their questions, be clear in your answers."

An experienced hiker and writer, author Tom Watson has selected 60 of the best hikes in and around the Twin Cities metropolitan area. From urban hikes that make use of parklands and streets to flora-and-fauna-rich treks along the Mississippi to aerobic outings along the area's glaciated hills, Watson provides hikers (and walkers) with a great variety of hikes—and all within roughly 60 miles of Minneapolis and St. Paul.

You'll get more out of this book if you take a moment to read the Introduction explaining how to read the trail listings. The "Topographic Maps" section will help you understand how useful topos will be on a hike, and will also tell you where to get them. And though this is a "where-to," not a "how-to" guide, those of you who have not hiked extensively will find the Introduction of particular value.

As much for the opportunity to free the mind as to free the body, let Tom Watson's hikes elevate you above the urban hurry.

All the best.
The editors at Menasha Ridge Press

Preface

So Many Options

Within the seven county "metro" area that encompasses the Twin Cities of Minneapolis and St. Paul lies a network of literally hundreds of miles of trails. In the state of 10,000 lakes, nearly 1,000 of them lie within these urban borders. Consequently, Minneapolis was dubbed the "City of Lakes". Once you discover all the trails throughout this same area, you may be inclined to call the Twin Cities " The Cities of Trails"!

Some of these trails are broad, paved corridors through multi-use parks generously developed to provide myriad recreational opportunities for the young and old, the robust trekker and the casual stroller. Other trails are country lanes, walkways of grass winding through majestic stands of Minnesota hardwoods. Still others are a spider-web networks that remind one of well-used deer trails.

Some are isolated within a pocket of greenery surrounded by vast ribbons of freeway concrete and broad subdivisions. Others are woven within the fabric of parklands so expansive that you could literally spend weeks hiking all the networks lying within their folds.

The Trails Included

Where ever there was a network of trails, I tried to pick a trail that was representative of the area —those that showcased the park or region's main attractions or personality. As you find certain areas more appealing, you will also find other trails that you feel are more exciting or more challenging. That's the beauty of exploration and discovery. The trails cited in this guidebook are offered to introduce you to a particular hike and let your own wanderlust take it from there.

I deliberately chose not to include the regional corridors that are part of this vast system of trails. These are wonderful pathways—the Luce Line Trail that bisects the entire western region of the Twin Cities,

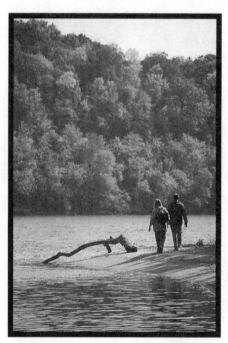

A couple walking along the Mississippi River.

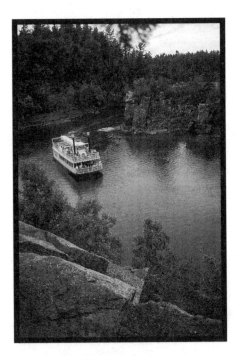

A paddlewheel boat on the St. Croix River at Interstate Dells.

the Hennepin Regional Trails, and the Scott County Regional Trail—many sections of which were reclaimed from discarded railroad right-of-ways. They are primarily bike corridors upon which you can also hike. They are great for connecting one park to another via greenbelts or low-traffic routes. I consider these the interstates and freeways of the hiking world. The trails covered in this book are more the back roads and neighborhood routes that really showcase the areas through which they pass.

A Few Considerations

Most of the trail descriptions are self explanatory. I am a moderate-paced hiker. I enjoy looking off the trial to the side. I carry binoculars, as I am an avid birder. I also carry a camera and an appropriate lens combination for both scenic shots and close-ups of flowers and insects.

The maps have been produced either from those available at the park's visitor center or at a trailhead or kiosk information unit. Sometimes these maps don't quite offer as much information as you discover en route, particularly at intersections and path options. I've tried to fix most of those omissions. Common sense and a bit of dead reckoning should keep you well oriented. If you stay on the main trail it's nearly impossible to become lost.

Some of the trails you'll encounter are multi-use (hiking and biking) trails by design. Sharing the route with cyclists means respecting their right-of-ways as you would hope they respect yours. On some of the hikes, pedestrian and bike "lanes" are separated by subtle barriers or restraints, on others traffic is married onto the same pathway for the entire route. Be extra cautious at turns and hills; be courteous; be safe.

Some of the trailheads for these hikes are heavily trafficked and others far less so, but theft is an unfortunate possibility at all of them. When you leave your car at a trailhead, park it well away from the road in order to reduce the likelihood of a collision and be sure to lock it. Leave your valuables out of sight and don't tempt thieves with rolled-down widows. The risks of theft and vandalism are minimal, but there's no reason not to take simple precautions that minimize them further.

Get Out There

The descriptions in this guidebook profile trails ranging from a paved sidewalk around a neighborhood lake to former railroad grades to narrow paths along the banks of the mighty Mississippi River. They were chosen to include specific trails that best showcase the type and quality of natural or historical amenities within a park or area. Each hike opens the door to other possibilities within the same network of trails.

I encourage readers to use the information herein as a starting point to get to know a park or primitive area. Use this book like a menu, choose the hike that suits your tastes for a sample of the trail entrées each park has to offer. The portions are all within a day's range of hiking and the bounty is quite fulfilling.

Hiking Recommendations

Note: Numbers corresponds to hike locations map on pages viii–ix.

Hikes 3 miles or less

2 Ann Lake, Sand Dunes State Forest
4 Barn Bluff
5 Bass Pond Trail, Long Meadow Lake
8 Bryant Lake Figure Eight
11 Clifton E. French Regional Park
12 Coon Rapids Dam
13 Cottage Grove Ravine Regional Park
14 Crosby Farm Park
18 Fish Lake Regional Park
20 Frontenac State Park (Bluffside Trail)
21 Hay Creek (West Trail)
22 Hyland Lakes Reserve (Richardson Interpretive Trail)
26 Lake Byllesby Regional Park
27 Lake Como, Como Park
30 Lake Minnewashta (Marsh Trail Loop)
31 Lake Nokomis
35 Lebanon Hills State Park (Holland/Jensen Lakes Loop)
36 Long Lake
39 Minnehaha Falls and Creek
41 Murphy-Hanrehan Park Reserve
46 Rice Creek Chain of Lakes Regional Park Reserve
47 Rice Lake State Park
48 Rum River Central
50 Sakatah Lake State Park
53 Spring Lake Park Reserve (Schaar's Bluff Trail)
54 Tamarack Nature Center
55 Tamarack Trail, Lowry Nature Center-Carver Park Reserve
56 Thompson Trail, Thompson County Park
60 Wood Lake Nature Center

Hikes more than 3 and less than 5 miles

1 Afton State Park
6 Battle Creek
7 Baylor Regional Park
10 Cleary Lake Regional Park
15 Crow-Hassen Regional Park
16 Eastman Nature Trail
23 Interstate Park, Minnesota
24 Interstate Park, Wisconsin
25 Kinnickinnic State Park
28 Lake Elmo Park Reserve, Eagle Point Lake
29 Lake Maria State Park
32 Lake Phalen
34 Lawrence Trail, Minnesota Valley
37 Mazomani Trail, Louisville Swamp/ Minnesota Valley
38 Miesville Ravine Park
42 Nerstrand Woods State Park (Big Woods Trail)
44 Pine Point Park Trail
49 Rum River North
52 Snail Lake
57 Wild River
58 William O'Brien State Park (Upper Park Trail)
59 Willow River, Wisconsin

Hikes more than 5 and less than 10 miles

3 Baker Park Reserve
19 Fort Snelling State Park (Snelling Lake and Pine Island Trails)
33 Lake Rebecca
40 Mississippi Gorge Trail
43 Old Cedar Avenue Trail, Long Meadow Lake
59 Sherburne NWR (Prarie's Edge Trail)

Hikes more than 10 miles long
9   City Lakes Chain, Lakes Harriet, Calhoun, and Isles
17 Elm Creek Park Reserve
45 Red Cedar Trail

Hikes on flat terrain
5   Bass Pond Trail, Long Meadow Lake
7   Baylor Regional Park
9   City Lakes Chain, Lakes Harriet, Calhoun, and Isles
10 Cleary Lake Regional Park
12 Coon Rapids Dam
14 Crosby Farm Park
17 Elm Creek Park Reserve
19 Fort Snelling State Park (Snelling Lake and Pine Island Trails)
25 Kinnickinnic State Park, Wisconsin
26 Lake Byllesby Regional Park
27 Lake Como, Como Park
28 Lake Elmo Park Reserve, Eagle Point Lake
31 Lake Nokomis
32 Lake Phalen
33 Lake Rebecca
34 Lawrence Trail, Minnesota Valley
36 Long Lake
40 Mississippi Gorge Trail
43 Old Cedar Avenue Trail, Long Meadow Lake
44 Pine Point Park Trail
45 Red Cedar Trail
46 Rice Creek Chain of Lakes Regional Park Reserve
47 Rice Lake State Park
48 Rum River Central
49 Rum River North
51 Sherburne NWR (Prarie's Edge Trail)
52 Snail Lake
53 Spring Lake Park Reserve (Schaar's Bluff Trail)
54 Tamarack Nature Center
55 Tamarack Trail, Lowry Nature Center-Carver Park Reserve
60 Wood Lake Nature Center

Hikes on hilly terrain
1   Afton State Park
2   Ann Lake, Sand Dunes State Forest
4   Barn Bluff
6   Battle Creek
13 Cottage Grove Ravine Regional Park
20 Frontenac State Park (Bluffside Trail)
21 Hay Creek (West Trail)
22 Hyland Lakes Reserve (Richardson Interpretive Trail)
24 Interstate Park, Wisconsin
29 Lake Maria State Park
30 Lake Minnewashta (Marsh Trail Loop)
35 Lebanon Hills State Park (Holland/Jensen Lakes Loop)
39 Minnehaha Falls and Creek
41 Murphy-Hanrehan Park Reserve
42 Nerstrand Woods State Park (Big Woods Trail)
58 William O'Brien State Park (Upper Park Trail)
59 Willow River, Wisconsin

Hikes on multi-use trails
3   Baker Park Reserve
6   Battle Creek
7   Baylor Regional Park
8   Bryant Lake Figure Eight
10 Cleary Lake Regional Park
18 Fish Lake Regional Park
19 Fort Snelling State Park (Snelling Lake and Pine Island Trails)
27 Lake Como, Como Park
32 Lake Phalen
36 Long Lake
40 Mississippi Gorge Trail
43 Old Cedar Avenue Trail, Long Meadow Lake
45 Red Cedar Trail, Wisconsin
46 Rice Creek Chain of Lakes Regional Park Reserve
48 Rum River Central
49 Rum River North
51 Sherburne NWR (Prarie's Edge Trail)

Hikes suitable for young children
5   Bass Pond Trail, Long Meadow Lake
7   Baylor Regional Park
10 Cleary Lake Regional Park
12 Coon Rapids Dam
16 Eastman Nature Trail
26 Lake Byllesby Regional Park

27 Lake Como, Como Park
31 Lake Nokomis
32 Lake Phalen
36 Long Lake
42 Nerstrand Woods State Park (Big Woods Trail)
60 Wood Lake Nature Center

Hikes with interesting or abundant flora

1   Afton State Park
2   Ann Lake, Sand Dunes State Forest
16 Eastman Nature Trail
17 Elm Creek Park Reserve
20 Frontenac State Park (Bluffside Trail)
42 Nerstrand Woods State Park (Big Woods Trail)

Hikes good for bird-watching

1   Afton State Park
3   Baker Park Reserve
5   Bass Pond Trail, Long Meadow Lake
12 Coon Rapids Dam
35 Lebanon Hills State Park (Holland/Jensen Lakes Loop)
43 Old Cedar Avenue Trail, Long Meadow Lake
58 William O'Brien State Park (Upper Park Trail)
59 Willow River, Wisconsin
60 Wood Lake Nature Center

Hikes showcasing fall foliage

1   Afton State Park
3   Baker Park Reserve
4   Barn Bluff
13 Cottage Grove Ravine Regional Park
14 Crosby Farm Park
15 Crow-Hassen Regional Park
20 Frontenac State Park (Bluffside Trail)
21 Hay Creek (West Trail)
23 Interstate Park, Minnesota
29 Lake Maria State Park
35 Lebanon Hills State Park (Holland/Jensen Lakes Loop)

37 Mazomani Trail, Louisville Swamp/ Minnesota Valley
38 Miesville Ravine Park
39 Minnehaha Falls and Creek
42 Nerstrand Woods State Park (Big Woods Trail)
44 Pine Point Park Trail
53 Spring Lake Park Reserve (Schaar's Bluff Trail)

Hikes featuring historical sites

2   Ann Lake, Sand Dunes State Forest
4   Barn Bluff
5   Bass Pond Trail, Long Meadow Lake
12 Coon Rapids Dam
14 Crosby Farm Park
19 Fort Snelling State Park (Snelling Lake and Pine Island Trails)
20 Frontenac State Park (Bluffside Trail)
21 Hay Creek (West Trail)
34 Lawrence Trail, Minnesota Valley
37 Mazomani Trail, Louisville Swamp/ Minnesota Valley
39 Minnehaha Falls and Creek
40 Mississippi Gorge Trail
42 Nerstrand Woods State Park (Big Woods Trail)
43 Old Cedar Avenue Trail, Long Meadow Lake

Special geographic features

4   Barn Bluff
20 Frontenac State Park (Bluffside Trail)
23 Interstate Park, Minnesota
24 Interstate Park, Wisconsin
34 Lawrence Trail, Minnesota Valley
37 Mazomani Trail, Louisville Swamp/ Minnesota Valley
39 Minnehaha Falls and Creek
40 Mississippi Gorge Trail
42 Nerstrand Woods State Park (Big Woods Trail)
43 Old Cedar Avenue Trail, Long Meadow Lake
45 Red Cedar Trail, Wisconsin
59 Willow River, Wisconsin

Introduction

60 Hikes Within 60 Miles: Twin Cities, as the title suggests, offers hikers a descriptive glimpse of some of the best day-hiking trails within an hour's drive of downtown Minneapolis and St. Paul, Minnesota's Twin Cities. Interconnecting trail networks enable hikers to literally walk from one end of the metropolitan area to the other, all the while enjoying pockets of flora and fauna that might otherwise go unnoticed, including preserved or restored pre-settlement prairies and northern forests.

If you're new to hiking or even if you're a seasoned trailsmith, take a few minutes to read the following introduction. We explain how this book is organized and how to use it, better enabling you to access the many splendid trail miles that await.

Hike Profiles

Each listing has six key items: a locator map, an In Brief description, an At-a-Glance Information box, directions to the trailhead, a trail map, and a narrative hike description. Combined, these elements provide the means to assess each trail from the comfort of your favorite chair.

Locator Map

After narrowing down the general area of the hike on the overview map (see pages viii–ix), use the locator map, along with driving directions given in the profile, to find the trailhead. At the trailhead, park only in designated areas.

In Brief

This synopsis of the trail offers a snapshot of what to expect along the trail, including mention of historical sights, beautiful vistas, or other interesting sights you may encounter.

At-a-Glance Information

The At-a-Glance Information boxes give you a quick idea of the specifics of each hike. There are 13 basic elements covered:

Length The length of the trail from start to finish. There may be options to shorten or extend the hikes, but the mileage corresponds to the described hike and hike map. Consult the hike description to help decide how to customize the hike for your ability or time constraints.

Configuration A description of what the trail might look like from overhead. Trails can be loops, out-and-backs (that is, along the same route), or figure eights, or any of those in modified form. Sometimes the descriptions might surprise you.

Difficulty The degree of effort an "average" hiker should expect on a given hike. I have used familiar terms and explained in the Preface his personal preference for liesurely hiking.

Scenery Summarizes the overall environs of the hike and what to expect in terms of terrain and land use

Exposure A quick check of how much sun you can expect on your shoulders during the hike. Descriptive terms used are self-explanatory and include terms such as shady, exposed, and sunny.

Traffic Indicates how busy the trail might be on an average day. Trail traffic, of course, will vary from day to day and season to season.

Trail surface Indicates whether the trail is paved, rocky, smooth dirt, or a mixture of elements.

Hiking time How long it took the author to hike the trail.

Access Notes times of day when hike route is open, days on which it is officially closed, and when fees or permits are needed to access the trail.

Maps Which maps are useful in the author's opinion, for this hike and where to find them.

Facilities Notes any facilities such as rest rooms, phones, and water available at the trailhead or on the trail or nearby.

Special comments Provides you with those little extra details that don't fit into any of the above categories. Here you'll find reminders about such matter as park or road gate closings that could trap you or your car, trails that are susceptible to flooding, and hunting seasons that could affect your hiking.

Directions

Check here for directions to the trailhead. Used with the locator map, the directions will help you locate each trailhead.

Description

The trail description is the heart of each hike. Here, the author has provided a summary of the trail's essence as well as highlighted any special traits the hike offers. Ultimately the hike description will help you choose which hikes are best for you.

Nearby Activities

Look here for information on nearby din-

ing, recreational opportunities, or other activities to fill out your day.

Weather

Minnesota's weather makes no exceptions for the Twin Cities. It can make you unsuspectingly confident of sunshine and warmth or a worried second-guesser, all within a matter of hours. Dressing in layers is always a good plan. Even during spectacularly sunny weather, bringing a waterproof windbreaker is good comfort insurance against a cool lake breeze or persistent drizzle from a renegade rain cloud.

Four distinct seasons, each with attitude, present almost every form of weather imaginable through the course of a year.

Hiking in the Twin Cities can be done year-round on many of the trails, most of the time. Exceptions are unseasonably cold or excessively snowy weather. Some summer hiking trails are switched over to cross-country skiing routes when winter sets in. Other trails can be used for winter hiking and snowshoeing.

While most trails mentioned in this book offer their amenities and attractions throughout the season, those that are particularly enjoyable during a certain season are noted in their profiles.

Early spring and late fall are especially nice times to hike in areas with dense understory, because less foliage means you can see deeper into the woods. Of course, hiking under a the thick summer canopy of lush leaves or strolling through flaming fall colors is cause enough to hike these trails several times a year.

Average Daily (High/Low) Temperatures by Month, Twin Cities, Minnesota

Month	High	Low
January	20	2
February	26	9

March	39	22
April	56	36
May	69	47
June	78	57
July	84	63
August	80	60
September	70	50
October	58	38
November	41	25
December	25	10

Average lows and highs range from 2°F to 20°F in January to 63°F to 84°F and higher in July. The heaviest monthly rainfall occurs between May (above 2") and September (above 2.5"), peaking at about 4" in July. The average humidity for this region between May and September is about 53%.

Ecological Regions

There are three main ecological regions in Minnesota: northern conifers (also called "Pinelands"), hardwood forests, and prairies. Two of these regions, the Pinelands and hardwoods, converge very close to the Twin Cities. Many of the Twin Cities area parks feature the aspen, birch, spruce, and fir forests that make up the main species of the Pinelands region. Coupled with the lakes, bogs, and wildlife associated with such regions, these parks offer hikers an opportunity to experience the type of ecological flora and fauna common to the state's northern regions.

The prairies of Minnesota, which once covered vast portions of Minnesota and millions of acres of the Great Plains, are now preserved in small sections and plots through this region. Many of the hikes in this book include routes through or around re-established prairie systems within a park or preserve.

Area Geology

There are four main geological areas that converge at the Twin Cities: The "Big Woods" of mixed hardwoods that virtually covered the eastern half of Minnesota before settlements encroached from the east. These dominate the western portions of the Twin Cities as well as a few major remnants to the south. The St. Croix moraines are glacial deposits left over from the last Ice Age. Much of the landscape east of St. Paul has been sculpted into reminders of the great sheet of ice that once covered the area. To the north of the Twin Cities lie the great sand plains of Anoka. Jack pine forests dominate this area. The oak savannas of the southern portion of the Twin Cities region are reminders of the vastness of the prairies and plains that once covered the entire midwest. The savannahs with their rolling hills, island of oaks and other hardwoods, and pockets of open prairie-like cover are slowly being brought back in many of the parks through prairie restoration projects, some of which are mentioned in association with particular hikes in this book.

Coupled with the lakes, bogs and wildlife associated with such regions, these parks offer hikers an opportunity to experience the type of ecological flora and fauna characteristic of this region of Minnesota.

Maps

The maps in this book have been produced with great care and, when used with the hiking directions, will help you get to the trailhead and stay on course. But as any experienced hiker knows, things can get tricky off the beaten path.

For even more information on a particular trail look to the United States Geological Survey's 7.5 minute series topographic maps (topos). Recognizing how indispensable these are to hikers, many outdoor shops now carry topos of the local area.

If you're new to hiking, you might be wondering, "What's a topographic map?" In short, topos indicate not only linear distance but elevation as well. One glance at a topo will show you the difference: Contour lines spread across the map like dozens of intricate spider webs. Each contour line represents a particular elevation, and at the base of each topo a particular contour interval designation is given.

Let's assume that the 7.5 minute series topo reads "Contour Interval 40 feet," that the short trail we'll be hiking is 2 inches in length on the map, and that it crosses 5 contour lines from its beginning to end. What do we know? Well, because the linear scale of this series is 2,000 feet to the inch (roughly 2.75 inches representing one mile), we know our trail is approximately 0.8 miles long (2 inches are 2,000 feet). But we also know we'll be climbing or descending 200 vertical feet (5 contour lines at 40 feet each) over that distance. And the elevation designations written on occasional contour lines will tell us if we're heading up or down.

In addition to outdoor shops and bike shops, other places in the Twin Cities metro area likely to carry topos are major universities and some public libraries, where you may be able to photocopy the ones you need to avoid the cost of buying them

Trail Etiquette

Whether you're on a city walk or on a long hike, remember that great care and resources (from nature as well as from tax dollars) have gone into creating the trails and paths. Taking care of them begins with you, the hiker. Treat the trail, wildlife, flora, and your fellow hikers with respect. Here are a few general ideas to keep in mind while hiking:

1. Hike on open trails only. Respect trail and road closures (ask if you're not sure), avoid trespassing on private land, and obtain any required permits or authorization. Leave gates as you found them or as marked.

2. Leave no trace of your visit other than footprints. Be sensitive to the land beneath your feet. This also means staying on the trail and not creating any new trails. Be sure to pack out what you pack in. No one likes to see trash someone else has left behind.

3. Never spook animals. Give animals extra room and time to adjust to you.

4. Plan ahead. Know your equipment, your ability, and the area in which you are hiking—and prepare accordingly. Be self-sufficient at all times; carry necessary supplies for changes in weather or other conditions. A well-executed trip is a satisfaction to you and not a burden or offense to others.

5. Be courteous to other hikers, bikers, and all other people you meet while hiking.

Water

"How much is enough? One bottle? Two? Three?! But think of all that extra weight!" Well, one simple physiological fact should convince you to err on the side of excess when it comes to deciding how much water to pack: While working hard in 90° heat, we each need approximately 10 quarts of fluid every day. That's 2.5 gallons—12 large water bottles or 16 small ones. And, with water weighing in at approximately 8 pounds per gallon, a 1-day supply comes to a whopping 20 pounds.

In other words, pack along one or two bottles even for short hikes. Most—but not all—of the hikes in this book have water at the trailhead or along the way. But if you must use water that's not from a tap, make sure you purify it. If you drink it untreated, you run the risk of disease.

Many hikers pack along the inexpensive and only slightly distasteful tetraglycine hydroperiodide purification tablets (sold under the names Potable Aqua, Globaline, and Coughlan's, among others). Time for these tablets to work their magic is usually about 30 minutes—the colder the water, the longer it takes. Some invest in portable, lightweight purifiers that filter out the crud. Unfortunately, even the best filters only remove up to 98–99% of all those nasty bacteria, viruses, and other organisms you can't see.

Tablets or iodine drops by themselves will knock off the well-known Giardia. One to four weeks after ingestion, Giardia will have you bloated, vomiting, shivering with chills, and living in the bathroom.

But there are other parasites to worry about, including cryptosporidium. "Crypto" brings on symptoms very similar to Giardia, but unlike that fellow protozoan it's equipped with a shell sufficiently strong to protect it against the chemical killers that stop Giardia cold. This means either boiling the water or using a water filter to screen out both Giardia and crypto, plus the iodine to knock off viruses.

Some water filters come equipped with an iodine chamber to guarantee nearly full protection. Or you can simply add a pill or drops to the water you've just filtered (if you aren't allergic to iodine, of course). The pleasures of hiking—and the displeasure of getting sick—make this relatively minor effort worth every one of the few minutes involved.

Nasty Plants

Poison ivy is ever present in the region's forested parks. It can be a small, unimposing bush or a taller, shrub-like bush. Learning to recognize it by its distinct three-lobed compound leaf will reward you many times over during the summer and fall.

Another nasty plant, stinging nettle, can produce a burn similar to that of a jellyfish or other vile skin irritating plants and animals. Learn to identify this tall, tooth-edged leafy plant as well.

While several species of shrubs, such as the woody hawthorn and the more vine-like raspberry, have thorns, none compare to the prickly mountain ash. Unassuming as it grows along the trail, looking innocently like a small green ash, the prickly ash has needle-sharp thorns ready to bite the hand that grabs it or lash out at an arm or leg that passes too closely.

First-Aid Kit

A typical kit may contain more items than you might think necessary. These are just the basics:

Sunscreen
Aspirin or acetaminophen
Butterfly-closure bandages
Band-Aids
Snakebite kit
Gauze (one roll)
Gauze compress pads (a half-dozen 4" x 4")
Ace bandages or Spenco joint wraps
Benadryl or the generic equivalent—diphenhydramine (an antihistamine, in case of allergic reactions)
A prefilled syringe of epinephrine (for those known to have severe allergic reactions to such things as bee stings)
Water purification tablets or water filter (on longer hikes)
Moleskin or Spenco "Second Skin"
Hydrogen peroxide or iodine
Antibiotic ointment (Neosporin or the generic equivalent)
Matches or pocket lighter
Whistle (more effective in signaling rescuers than your voice)

Pack the items in a waterproof bag such as a Ziploc bag or a similar product.

What to Wear

Proper foot gear is absolutely essential. Griping soles and solid ankle support are mandatory—even on groomed or paved pathways. A properly worn-in boot or hiking shoe should be used, especially on longer hikes. Breaking in a stiff pair of trekking shoes on even a 5-mile hike can breed a crop of blisters.

Whether you should wear long pants or shorts is a personal preference and one based on whether you expect to bush-whack your way through a park. Some trails lead through sensitive areas and you are requested to stay on the path. Other areas, however, almost draw the hiker off the path and into the woods.

What to Bring

Besides a camera bag, none of these trails should necessitate carrying anything more than a fanny pack or day pack. Adequate water for your metabolism and thirst-quenching needs should be carried at all times. Most of the areas provide water, either at the trailhead, along some trails or at the visitor center/park headquarters.

Fuel, in the form of snacks—energy bars, trail mix—is a personal preference. Person-ally, I like the idea of stopping at a particu-larly scenic overlook along a trail and having a snack while my other senses feast on all the stimuli surrounding me.

Most importantly, from my perspective anyway, is to bring along a notebook or journal to record what you see, sketch what you observe and describe what you think or feel along the trail. This and a good guidebook can expand your level of appre-ciation for all that surrounds you during each hike.

Hiking with Children

No one is too young for a nice hike in the woods or through a city park. Parents with infants can strap the little ones on with devices such as the Baby-Björn Baby Car-rier® or Kelty's Kangaroo®. Be careful, though. Flat, short trails are probably best with an infant. Toddlers who have not quite mastered walking can still tag along, riding on an adult's back in a child carrier.

Children who are walking can, of course, follow along with an adult. Use common sense to judge a child's capacity to hike a particular trail. Always plan for the possibility that the child will tire quickly and have to be carried. When packing for the hike, remember the child's needs as well as your own. Make sure children are adequately clothed for the weather, have proper shoes, and are proper-ly protected from the sun with sunscreen and clothing. Kids dehydrate quickly, so make sure you have plenty of clean water or other drinks for everyone.

Depending on age, ability, and the hike difficulty, most children should enjoy some of the short hikes described in this book. To assist an adult with determining which trails are suitable for children, a short list of hike recommendations for children is pro-vided on pages [xvi-xvii].

The Business Hiker

Whether you're in the Twin Cities area on business as a resident or visitor, these hikes are the perfect opportunity to make a quick getaway from the demands of com-merce. Some of the hikes are located close to government buildings and other office areas classified as urban and are easily acces-sible from downtown areas.

Instead of a burger down the street, pack a lunch and head for a nearby trail—the local and state parklands are a good bet—to take a relaxing break from the office or that tiresome convention. Or plan ahead and take along a small group of your business comrades. A well-planned half-day getaway is the perfect complement to a business stay in the Twin Cities metropolitan area.

Enjoy the Experience

What all these trails have in common is an opportunity to turn a part of your day into a "stroll in the park" right smack dab in the middle of the city. For some of us, a hike is a brisk walk for exercise, for others it's a leisurely-paced traipse through unex-plored woods. Sometimes it's a planned trek of discovery hoping perhaps to add a new bird to your life list or catch your favorite wildflower at peak bloom. Whatever the inspiration, the trails in this book are pathways to other activities, observations, and pleasures.

Of course, don't litter and don't remove things that others might enjoy. Collect images mentally or with a camera or sketch pad. Whether yours is the path less taken or the one deeply worn—enjoy each as though you were the first to lay foot upon it.

60 Hikes Within 60 Miles:

TWIN CITIES

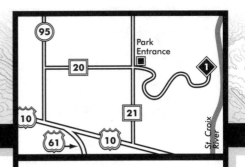

#1

Afton State Park

IN BRIEF

More than 20 miles of trails crisscross oak savannas and follow ravines cut deeper than 300 feet into the bluffs of the St. Croix River. This park provides hikers with serious trails, expansive river beaches, and myriad vistas of the beautiful St. Croix river and valley.

DIRECTIONS

From downtown St. Paul, head east on Interstate 94 for 9 miles to County Road 15. Go south 7 miles to Military Road (CR 20). Turn east and continue 3 miles to the park entrance. Drive to the Interpretive Center and park. The trail starts at the north end of parking lot.

DESCRIPTION

The main trail leaving from the parking lot at Afton Park is like a promenade leading to the main activity areas of the park. Its wide, paved path leads hikers down an incline along a gradually winding trail past the picnic area and group sites atop a wooded ridge above the river. The ridge-top trail ends at a series of steps that drops the trail quickly to the lowlands along the river. There it continues through lowland forests of spindly maples, ironwoods, ash, and a dense understory. The trail crosses an unnamed creek (great for wading in on those hot, humid days of summer) and opens onto the main path, an old railroad grade that serves as the main trail

KEY AT-A-GLANCE INFORMATION

Length: 4.3 miles

Configuration: Balloon

Difficulty: Moderate to strenuous due to elevation changes exceeding 300 feet in less than 0.5 mile; easy along upper meadows and lowlands

Scenery: Mature oak forests, delicate prairies, ravines, and impressive vistas of the St. Croix river

Exposure: Fully exposed meadows atop bluffs; dense canopies in ravines

Traffic: Popular with hikers, beaches get crowded in summer

Trail Surface: Paved surface, wide grassy lanes, and narrow, uneven surfaces along ravines

Hiking Time: 2 hours

Season: All season; many trails are converted for cross-country skiing

Access: Minnesota State Park fee system—$4 daily, $20 annual permit, or $12 annual permit for disabled individuals

Maps: Available at park or at www.dnr.state.mn.us/ parks_and_ recreation/state_parks/afton

Facilities: Developed campsites, picnic areas, rest rooms, beach, and interpretive center

Special Comments: This park is great for weekend campers/hikers

1

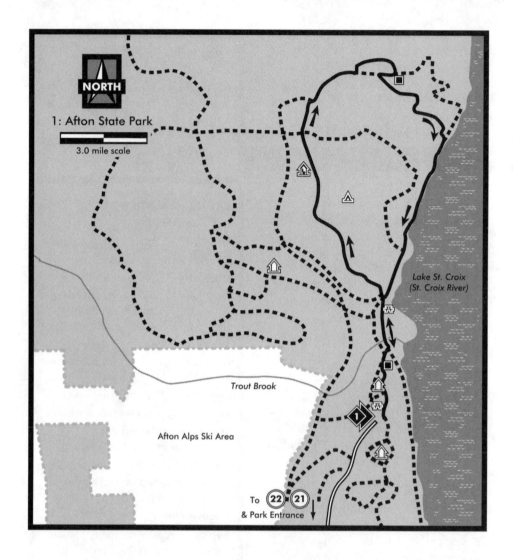

Lake St. Croix
(St. Croix River)

Trout Brook

Afton Alps Ski Area

To ㉒ ㉑
& Park Entrance

along the river, before bringing trekkers onto the lower picnic and beach area along the St. Croix River.

At this intersection, hiking trails weave out to the north and west to join up with a spider web of trails in the northern region of Afton Park.

If you take the trail to the far left, you'll climb steep ravines to a savanna-like plateau encircled by trails. Major horseback riding trails and hiking trails depart from this meadow, cutting back

down through more ravines on the west end of the park to form a large looping network of trails.

Save those trails for another day, and instead head straight, along the trail leading up to the backpacker's camping area. The trail weaves uphill through stands of oak and maple. This trail leads to some of the highest points in the northern section of the park—with a rise of over two hundred feet in the first one-third of a mile. It's a gradual ascent with a turn-out observation point and rest stop that over-looks the ravine to the southwest.

Reaching the plateau, the trail levels off and opens up onto grassy corridors between islands of scrub oak and bushes. Numbered trail spurs lead off perpendicular from this trail to the dozen campsites scattered throughout the area. Lying off the trail and cut into the edge of the woods, campsites are fairly well hidden and obscured from view from the main trail.

A gravel trail, supplied firewood, toilets, and water (at campsite #10) provide nice amenities for campers. Remember this watering hole, its a great place to replenish containers. In summer, the meadows can get very warm, and there is no shade on the open bluff tops. Be sure to stay well hydrated and use sunscreen.

As the trail winds through the eastern edge of this meadow, vistas of the St. Croix valley become more accessible. The trail continues east, swinging back to the river at the end of the camping area. There is a small stand of pines just before a grassy field on a short, 0.3-mile loop (it's marked with a sign post). Early morning hikers might stand a good chance of glimpsing deer, foxes, and badgers in this area.

The trail continues on through a stand of cedars before coming to a good view across the river eastward into Wisconsin. This loop joins back into the main "campground" loop at a point labeled as a second watering hole on older maps. However, its been a few seasons since this hand pump has seen any action. If you think you'll run dry before returning to the parking lot, better get your water back at campsite #10.

You'll still want to pass by this intersection, though, as there is a nice perch at the observation area right beyond the pump. Its vista features a grand view of the lower St. Croix before it joins the Mississippi River several miles downstream. This is also a good place to rest your legs before the steady 200-foot descent back down a ravine before hitting the river trail again.

The trail is hard-packed earth (clay-loam soil) and heads right down the side of the ravine without many twists or turns. These ravines are typical of many in this part of the state. Walking through this modest understory, you'll spy tree trunks grown tall and somewhat spindly from the extra strain to reach sunlight above. Typically, these ravines have seasonal flowages running down them. In early spring, these areas can be especially muddy because of all the drainage patterns converging in them.

As you level out in the floodplain area of the river, you meet back up with the main river trail/bike corridor. Continuing on past this intersection allows you to step out onto the broad, sandy shoreline of the St. Croix. You can follow the rocky, sandy river bank back to the lower picnic/swimming area or just spend some moments cooling off below the massive cottonwood canopies that tower over the edge of the river. During the summer, there will be a constant regatta of pleasure boats cruising back and forth along the river from bend to bend.

If you backtrack from the river, you'll hit the broad roadway of the main trail that parallels the banks about fifty feet above the river. This pathway is lined with birch and oak trees. Several openings keep the river in view to the east of the trail.

A little over a half mile south, the trail brings hikers back to the swimming area and the intersection with the trail that leads back up to the parking lot. The railroad bed trail along the river continues on, extending south from the swimming area to the far southern corner of Afton Park.

The climb back up the 85 stairs may seem a bit strenuous after all the ravine hiking, so there is an alternate route via a 180° switchback trail just beyond the stairway. Both take you to the top and back out to the parking lot before the visitor center.

NEARBY ACTIVITIES

Summer hikers who are equally at home on a mountain bike as in hiking boots can bring their bikes or rent a bike next door at the Afton Ski Area, which doubles as a hilly mountain bike playground in the summer. Winter snowshoe-hikers can enjoy the same area for some of the best skiing in the metro area.

#2
Ann Lake, Sand Dunes State Forest

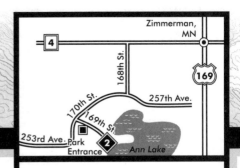

IN BRIEF

One of many in the Sand Dunes State Forest, this hiker-only trail wanders through Bob Dunn Recreation Area. It highlights white and red pine tree plantations and offers a good example of Minnesota's northern sandy soil country.

DIRECTIONS

Take US Highway 169 north from Minneapolis to Zimmerman, Minnesota. Take County Road 4 west (left) 4.5 miles past CR 15 to 168th Street. Take a left and go 0.2 mile to Dunes Forest Road. Turn right following the sign to Ann Lake. Drive 0.6 mile to the entrance of Bob Dunn Recreation Area on the left. Follow the road to the parking lot and picnic area.

DESCRIPTION

This hike lies in the midst of a greater natural/recreational area comprised of the Sherburne National Wildlife Refuge, Sand Dunes State Forest, and the Uncas Dunes Scientific and Nature Area. Multipurpose trails weave through the area. A representative hike in the Bob Dunn Recreation Area showcases the region over 3 miles of earthen paths.

Start at the end of the parking lot by the picnic area. The trailhead is to the right, across the road. The lake is just a few steps further on. Head up the trail into an area forested with oak, spruce, and red pine. The trail immediately

KEY AT-A-GLANCE INFORMATION

Length: 2 miles

Configuration: Elongated loop

Difficulty: Moderate to easy throughout with some short but steep inclines

Scenery: Plantations of white and red pine, oak-covered sandy ridges

Exposure: Mixed full sun and dense shade within the plantations

Solitude: Trail loops through northern, less developed, less trafficked area of park

Trail Surface: Sandy and hard-packed earthen trails throughout

Hiking Time: 1 hour

Season: All seasons—the pines are especially beautiful after a snowfall

Access: No fee

Maps: Available at information kiosk on site (Sand Dunes State Forest Trail Map)

Facilities: Campground, outhouse, picnic area, drinking water, beach, and swimming area

Special Comments: The sand country is quite different from the bedrock glaciated areas further east and south; stands of pines are a pleasant alternative from predominantly hardwood forests

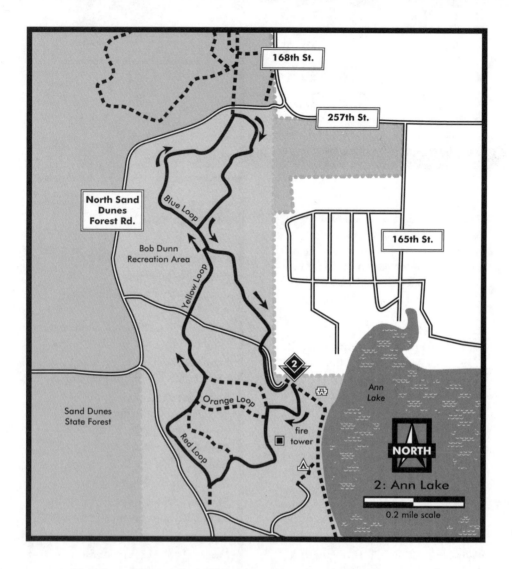

climbs a small, sandy knoll before taking a sharp right about 50 yards from the trailhead. This is a stretch of the Yellow Trail. You're on the right path if you come to an old hand-operated water pump on your left.

These sandy areas tend to produce solid stands of oak. The trail will meander through groves that combine red oak and pin oak trees. Young spruce seedlings, also part of the sandy soil ecology, have sprouted throughout this park. Just past the water pump, these seedlings,

some three or four feet tall, dominate the understory.

As you top the hill, there are views of the fire tower on your left. You can't climb it, but hilltop vistas reveal the surrounding park area over the tops of oaks below. You'll pass two intersections: the other end of the Yellow Loop and the beginning of the Orange Loop. Stay to the left past these two intersections. You will then be on the back half of the Orange Loop. This particular hike takes a clockwise course around the outer loops of the interconnecting color-coded trails (the area's trail maps are very accurate).

Just past the fire tower, the trail forks. The sandy path on the left drops down to a campsite, while the one to the right descends about 50 feet in elevation to continue the Orange Loop. At the bottom of the hill, you will come to yet another intersection. This is the Red Loop. Take it to the left.

The trail climbs uphill towards a white pine plantation. Notice a sign identifying poison ivy on the right. The short Red Loop follows the topography of the park around and through a stand of jack pine. Jack pine are a often seen sprouting up after forest fires. Their seed coat needs high temperatures to open. This length of the trail cuts close to the road before looping back around to the main trail. Keep to the right and take the trail as it climbs up into a stand of white pines. White pines have five, long, somewhat fine needles in a cluster. The white pine has a smoother, grayish bark as opposed to the red, scaly bark of the red pine.

As this trail cuts through the stand of white pines, notice the profusion of white pine seedlings scattered like weeds throughout the forest floor. This prolific growth of pines prompted successful plantation development in the 1940s, when the great depression saw farming in this sandy-soiled region suffer. Plantations may have helped stabilize the soil, which otherwise would have blown away. To date more than 2,400 acres of tree plantations have been established in the Sand Dunes State Forest. The majority of these grow pines, as on this trail.

A small cluster of jack pine, and a small aspen stand line the trail after the white pine plantation. Just beyond lie an open meadow area and yet another trail intersection. This is the Orange Loop again. Take the turn to the left. Now the trail rises in elevation to stands of older,

more mature oaks. You will also see a plantation of red pine. Notice the difference between these and the earlier whites? If not, you have a second chance. The trail next dips down into yet another white pine plantation before coming up on a ridge.

About two hundred yards beyond the intersection that brought you back onto the Orange Loop, the Orange Loop veers back to your right. Continue straight; this is the Yellow Loop again. Another 0.1 mile and you will cross over CR 254. You are now heading into the northern half of the recreation area. Another 0.15 mile, and you will come upon yet another trail intersection.

This is the Blue Loop, which is a 0.8 mile route through the northern quarter of the Bob Dunn Recreation Area. It continues its serpentine way up and down the sandy hills through varied forest types before coming back on itself. A left at the intersection continues through more mature oaks on the ridge. Again you will see more small white pines gaining a foothold on the ridge.

The trail cuts sharply to the right as it passes very near the park boundary. Soon the trail meets up with the main park entrance road and leads back to the parking lot where you began.

NEARBY ATTRACTIONS
The Ann Lake trail skirts the western edge of the lake. The southern portion is marshy, a good bird-viewing area. Also, at the north end of the park, connected to the Blue Loop, is another 0.5-mile loop, the Green Loop. For those seeking still more hiking options, there are corridors beyond the Blue Loop linking it to the North Orock Trail within Sand Dunes State Forest. These are multi-use trails open to hiking, walking, and snowmobiling.

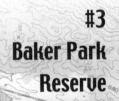

#3
Baker Park
Reserve

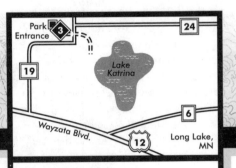

IN BRIEF

Woody highlands and evolving meadows and prairies are sprinkled throughout an otherwise marshy area around Lake Katrina. This 3,312-acre park reserve offers everything from golf and developed playgrounds to pathways skirting undeveloped marshlands.

DIRECTIONS

From west Minneapolis, take US Highway 12 west past Long Lake to County Road 29 (Baker Park Road). Turn right (north) and follow for about 1.4 miles to the park entrance on the left.

DESCRIPTION

Like other parks past the western edge of the Twin Cities metro area, Baker Park's 3,312 acres lie atop the Des Moines ground moraine, a remnant of the Wisconsin ice age, which covers this entire region. Its rolling topography, myriad ice-block lakes, and maple–basswood dominant forests are characteristics common to this part of Minnesota. Yet, like all other parks, Baker offers up its own personality to the intrepid hiker along its paved hiking/biking trails.

The entrance to the park is across the street from the actual trailhead, so park your vehicle and head back out the entrance and across Highway 29. You will see a trail spur on the right side of the roadway immediately upon entering that side of the park. Take this short,

KEY AT-A-GLANCE INFORMATION

Length: 6.2 miles

Configuration: Full circle

Difficulty: Flat and easy with a few gradual inclines

Scenery: A variety of forested areas, meadows, and only a brief glimpse of the lake

Exposure: Mostly full sun, some shade

Traffic: Popular trail for cyclists and runners, especially on weekends

Trail Surface: Paved

Hiking Time: 2–2½ hours

Season: All seasons (some trail segments converted to cross-country skiing in winter)

Access: $5 daily vehicle permit, $27 annual regional park permit

Maps: Available at park headquarters, or www.hennepinparks.org

Facilities: Campground, picnic area, rest rooms, pit toilets, boat rental, drinking water

Special Comments: Hiking/biking trail has faster bike traffic at times so be careful around corners and coming over rises in the trail

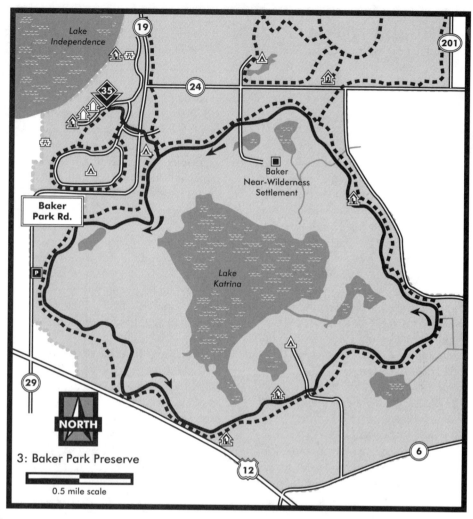

Baker Park Rd.

Lake Independence

Baker Near-Wilderness Settlement

Lake Katrina

NORTH

3: Baker Park Preserve

0.5 mile scale

paved spur down through a rather dense stand of trees to the **T** intersection. Take this trail to the right which will lead you through the entire southern half of the park. This trail, like other bike/hike loops, parallels the park's horse trail, but that trail is seldom visible and never crosses the hiking path.

You immediately pass through a representative sampling of the trees you can expect to see throughout the park: basswood, oak, cottonwoods, and elm (only the maples are missing in this section). On your left will be the marshy areas that surround Lake Katrina in the distance. The trail snakes through stands of sumac followed by open areas. Islands of trees are scattered along the modest hills upland from the lake.

At about 0.6 mile the trail cuts sharply to the right and climbs around a small pond. From there it continues toward more marshy areas a quarter mile farther. The trail finally straightens out a bit for the next 0.3 mile or so before coming to a trail spur to an alternate parking lot; here hikers and bikers can access the trail without going into the main part of the park.

I am not experienced enough to identify birds by their call, but I do recognize that different songs are from different birds, suggesting that Baker Park is a birder's challenge. For non-birders, the chorus of calls and chirps is ever present and delightful during the summer months.

As you continue along, you'll notice that the vegetation along the trail constantly changes from marsh to field to forest. After the parking lot, you'll encounter aspen and more sumac mixed in what appears to be second- or third-generation growth of forest species.

The terrain becomes wetter at about the 1.5-mile mark as indicated by islands of willows and more exposed vistas of the marshes and rush grass around the lake. All this will be on your left as you approach the boundary of the park and its proximity to US 12 just across the park's fenced border.

Shortly after leaving the fence behind, you'll get a good view of the lake. You will have hiked 2.5 miles at this point. The lake itself covers about 200 acres, while the boggy area surrounding it covers over 225 acres of marshland. Three tenths of a mile farther there is a picnic area and a rest room, all underneath a power line that crosses overhead.

The Katrina Camp entrance road soon comes up on the right at about 3 miles. This road has recently been made part of the access route that now joins Baker Park with the popular Luce Line Biking and Hiking Corridor, which runs extensively across the western reaches of the metro area.

The trail continues to wind around the southeastern edge of the lake, rising slowly from the marsh. You'll reach a rock bench at about 3.3 miles—a good resting point at about halfway along this trail. About a quarter mile farther, the trail drops down and passes a residential area bordering the park.

You'll come across a roadway leading left to the Trumpeter Swan Refuge. A resident flock of swans summers here, and around the third week of June the park offers an interpretive program featuring these local trumpeters.

For the next mile or so, check out all the maples—some of the stands are impressive with towering, dominant maples reminiscent of the "Big Woods" growth seen in other regions around the Twin Cities. Just past this stand of maples, the trail intersects with a path leading to the administration offices across CR 24. If you want to add 1.5 miles to the hike, you can access the short hiking-only figure-eight loop that begins at a spur by the administrative offices.

Staying on the main trail for another 0.3 mile will bring you past a shallow hillside with what appears to be an old landscape planting of both the indigenous and introduced plants that are currently scattered throughout the park. Another few tenths of a mile and the trail intersects the Baker Near Wilderness Settlement.

This is an experiential learning site for school-age children, special interest groups, and adult audiences. There are eight cabins that serve as a residential living environment for participants in the programs.

The road that intersects the trail crosses the highway and extends to the Marshview Group Camp. The road crosses the designated hiking trail that forms a figure-eight loop around the group camp and the area behind the administration building.

A bit further and the trail passes through a stand of box elders on the right. This is also a rest stop for hikers and horses. At this point you are about 6 miles along the trail. Watch the side of the trail closely for the sign for the Oak Knoll Group Camp. A very few yards past the Group Camp turn you'll come upon the unmarked spur on the right that takes you out of the thicker woods and back to the entrance.

NEARBY ACTIVITIES

Check with the park office for activities at the Near Wilderness Settlement or to get details on the hiking trail network behind the Administrative Office across County 24. With access now open to the Luce Line Trail Corridor, another 30 miles can be added to a determined trekker's agenda.

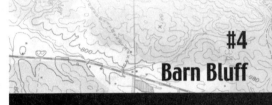

#4
Barn Bluff

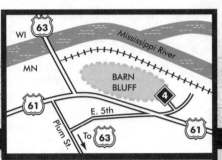

IN BRIEF

Coming into Red Wing from the north with the afternoon sun glowing on the sandstone walls of Barn Bluff is a sight worthy of the 45-minute drive south of the Cities. A landmark since people first trod the banks of the Mississippi River, Barn Bluff offers an invigorating ascent and spectacular views of the river valley and town below. The quick ascent via switchbacks to the base of the bluff, followed by a long stair climb to plateau, makes this a serious urban hike.

DIRECTIONS

From the Twin Cities, take US Highway 61 south from Hastings. Continue on US 61 through Red Wing to the south side of town. Barn Bluff looms ahead. Turn right at the last stop light and go to 5th Street. Turn left on 5th and follow it, first parallel to US 61 and then under highway overpass, to the parking area immediately on your right. The staircase to the trailhead is on the left, just across the street.

DESCRIPTION

"The most beautiful prospect that the imagination can form." That's how eighteenth-century explorer Jonathan Carver described the view from Barn Bluff. Rising 343 feet above the town of Red Wing, Barn Bluff still evokes similar feelings from many for whom it is a prospective climb. Henry David

KEY AT-A-GLANCE INFORMATION

Length: 1.75 miles

Configuration: Loop; random hiking once on top of bluff

Difficulty: Steep, can be treacherous in winter and late spring

Scenery: Birch- and maple-covered slopes plus an incredible 360° view of the Mississippi

Exposure: Mostly full sun at the top, shaded woods below

Traffic: Popular on bright, sunny days during summer

Trail Surface: Well-worn with exposed roots and rocks; very narrow in some places; on plateau, open grasses and some worn trails network along bluff top

Hiking Time: 1½–2½ hours

Season: Best from late spring through fall

Access: No fees, parking limited to narrow strip along street

Maps: None available other than interpretive map at trailhead

Facilities: None, although trailhead is at edge of residential and downtown districts

Special Comments: One of the best hikes in this area due to the view and the challenging riverside access

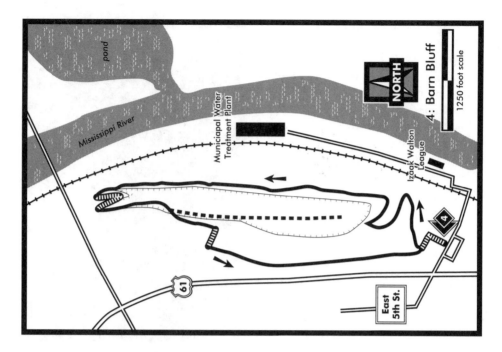

Thoreau probably agreed when he climbed it as a tourist. Stephen H. Long, the topographic engineer on an 1819 mapping expedition, no doubt found the prospect of the view from Barn Bluff alluring as well.

In the local Dakota tribal legends, the big bluff was the basis for a great tale. Two tribes fought over the "ownership" of the big bluff to such an extent that the Great Spirit is said to have split the massive rock in two so each tribe could have part of it. The other half is said to be Sugar Loaf down in Winona, about 60 miles downstream. The French named it La Grange, which translates "the barn." Hence, its more common name: Barn Bluff.

The bluff stands as a natural demarcation of the local geologic strata in the area. Glaciers carved deep channels around some of the more resistant formations, leaving huge islands in the inland sea created when ice thawed and retreated. A stratified history of the deposits is clearly exposed in the layers that make up Barn Bluff: Franconia green sandstone only 6–8 feet above the river, St. Lawrence dolestone (blue shale) for the next 45 feet up, Jordan sandstone (layers of white-yellow stone) for another 120 feet. These combine to form Barn Bluff's Cambrian layer, dated between 500 and 540 million years ago. A layer 75 feet thick of Prairie du Chien sandstone from the Ordovician period—500 to 440 million years ago—lies below the layer that caps the bluff—a relic of the Pleistocene era a mere 1.8 to 11,000 years ago. Some of these layers are exposed via erosion nearer the start of the climb, and later come into view as you climb up the bluff at just a dozen yards (in elevation) above the river.

To start this hike through geological history and personal prospecting, park at the turn-out just under the overpass for US 61. Climb the concrete staircase to the interpretive rest area to begin the actual trek around and up Barn Bluff.

I chose the path to the right. In late winter, with snow on the ground, this is a formidable path and can be very icy and unstable. However, it is the best trail to take for splendid river views, so pick your season.

The trail winds through an understory comprised mostly of oaks with some maple. This is a steady uphill climb over exposed ruts, irregular rocks, and narrow pathways. It continues up the south/easternmost end of the bluff. About 150 yards up the trail, just as you have a clear view over the edge to the river below and the Isaak Walton League clubhouse, there is a stone arch outlining a tunnel into the mountain. History buffs can scout out its purpose. It may be just an old storage chamber carved back into the wall. I'd question its safety and suggest you don't trespass. At this point you are nearing the base of the exposed rocky cap of the bluff and are about 75 feet above the river.

You come to an abrupt switchback that turns sharply to the left and back toward US 61. This portion of the trail is even steeper and narrower. It, too, is hazardous, with exposed rocks and more roots. The dominant trees are oak and birch with a honeysuckle understory. This curving, climbing trail takes you back to the highway side of the bluff and puts you right at the base of the rocks that cap Barn Bluff. The trail turns back again toward the river and continues north along the base of the rocks for the entire length of the bluff.

You'll primarily find birch trees on the north side of the bluff, with maples the second most common tree. The trail runs along the shoulder of relatively level ground between the bottom of the rocks and the steep descent to the river a couple hundred feet below. Railroad tracks parallel the base of the bluff, followed halfway around by a road that leads to

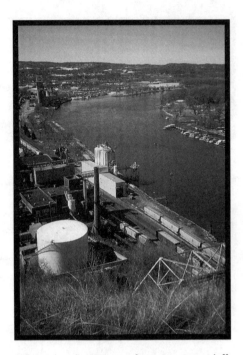

Industrial Red Wing seen from atop Barn Bluff.

the municipal water treatment facility. Immediately beyond the road is the bank of the river.

After traversing the length of the bluff, the trail heads back around the other side of the ridge just as the Eisenhower Bridge comes into view beyond the trees. The trail shrinks here and poses a few obstacles around fallen chunks of cliff side.

At the extreme northern end of the bluff is a set of concrete stairs, over 200 in all, that make a 180° switchback halfway up, to take hikers to the exposed cap of this great bluff. At the top of the stairs is a breathtaking view of downtown Red Wing, upriver on the Mississippi and across the Eisenhower Bridge into Wisconsin. Your prospecting imagination finally pays off when you look out over this platform at the head of those 200-plus steps.

The journey takes on a whole new hiking theme, as you can now walk casually up the slope some 30 feet more to be truly on top of the bluff. The vistas are remarkable, particularly to the south and west. A line of gnarly oaks and the whitest aspens I've ever seen grow along the eastern edge of the cap.

As you reach the top of the cap and look south along its entire length, there are two trails. One leads to the right; the other extends farther along the top of the cap. If you want to explore the summit, take the left trail and take your time, you could spend hours hiking the top. If you choose to retreat from the cap, choose the trail on the right. This takes you back to the west face of the bluff for the long, gradual descent to the interpretive rest area.

The trail begins as a gradual descent and then makes a sharp turn to the right and down yet another flight of concrete stairs, a drop about 50 feet over nine sets of six steps each. This is the alternate winter route that leads off from the left fork at the interpretive area. In late spring, this is the far safer route since it is exposed to the sun and much less icy and snow packed than the eastern face.

Once you descend the staircase, you'll find a trail to the right. This is a short loop to a secluded, local campfire area. There is also a narrow foot trail right along the base of the cliff that leads back to the first long stairway to the top. This is a much lesser-used trail, more dangerous than the designated routes shown on maps.

At the base of the stairs to the left is the long, gradual slope back down to the trailhead at the beginning. The trail cuts through a forested area of oaks and maples with moderate understory. This trail drops steadily for about 0.3 mile and will eventually level off as it meets up and runs parallel to US 61. A couple hundred yards further and the path returns to the first set of stairways you took up from the parking area.

NEARBY ACTIVITIES

The town of Red Wing is worth a day's visit. There are shops and restaurants, riverfronts, and historic buildings. You are not that far away from other hikes in the area: Frontenac, Miesville Ravine, and Hay Creek are all to the south—less than a half hour away.

#5
Bass Pond Trail, Long Meadow Lake

IN BRIEF

The Minnesota Valley National Wildlife Refuge is only 10 miles from downtown Minneapolis. That and its 34 miles of river bottoms teaming with wildlife and natural amenities make it one of only four urban wildlife refuges in the United States. In my book, it's one of the very best places to hike in the Twin Cities. Urban wildlife– and bird-watchers should put this on the top of their list of premiere viewing areas near Minneapolis and St. Paul.

DIRECTIONS

Entrance is located about 2 miles west of the Minnesota Valley National Wildlife Refuge Visitor Center. Take Interstate 494 to the 24th Avenue exit, turn south past the Mall of America and turn left (east) on East 86th Avenue. Follow 86th for about a block. As the road swings to the right, there is a sign on driveway to the left that leads to a parking lot at the gated entrance to the Bass Ponds.

DESCRIPTION

The Bass Ponds are fun to explore along their own half-mile hiking trail, and because its another 1.25 miles down to the Old Cedar Bridge Trail (and another 1.25 miles back) I've decided to describe these as the two distinct trails that they are. The best way to enjoy these trails may be to go out and hike to the other end of the trail and then retrace your steps back

KEY AT-A-GLANCE INFORMATION

Length: 3 miles (0.5-mile interpretive loop and 1.25 out-and-back)

Configuration: Balloon

Difficulty: Easy, mostly-level river-bottom trails, few rises; may be slippery during spring and summer

Scenery: Wide vistas over a large marshy/open-water lake; beautiful with early morning or evening sun

Exposure: Shaded along banks, sunny in meadow and marsh areas

Traffic: Single path along lake is less crowded than pond area; during the school year, the ponds are popular field classrooms for area schools

Trail Surface: Packed turf/earth

Hiking Time: 45–60 minutes for pond; 30 minutes to Old Cedar Ave.

Season: All seasons—snow shoes and skis during winter

Access: Small parking area at top before gate; no fees

Maps: Available at Refuge Headquarters off of I-494 and 34th Ave., and at Bass Ponds Environmental Study Area kiosk

Facilities: Parking, kiosk

Special Comments: The opportunity to connect with the Old Cedar Avenue trail is a bonus

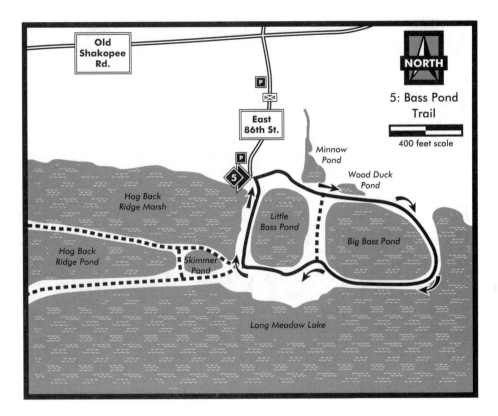

Old
Shakopee
Rd.

NORTH

5: Bass Pond
Trail

400 feet scale

East
86th St.

Minnow
Pond

Wood Duck
Pond

5

Hog Back
Ridge Marsh

Little
Bass Pond

Big Bass Pond

Hog Back
Ridge Pond

Skimmer
Pond

Long Meadow Lake

to the initial trailhead—rehiking the entire path and seeing things from the other direction.

A second option would be to put a shuttle vehicle at the opposite end of this trail so you don't have to retrace your route.

The gate to the Bass Ponds is always locked. Those with disabilities can get a key beforehand at the Refuge Visitor's Center. The roadway from the parking lot winds down into the lowlands. There, the river flats provide a nice transition from the suburban buzz of the freeway and residential neighborhood above.

Once you reach the bottom, you can obtain details about the area's historic and natural amenities from the information kiosk. Originally used by state officials as bass-rearing ponds back in the 1920s, this area was in operation for

more than 30 years. A spring-fed creek along the bottomlands provided the perfect aquatic conditions to create rearing ponds for over 2.5 million largemouth bass. New breeding ponds were added in 1938, at which time experiments to produce a cross between a musky and a northern pike were conducted. A hybrid was produced—one that grew so fast that it began cannibalizing its own whenever its standard food supply of minnows was not provided quickly.

Sunfish, crappie, and myriad other species were produced here and used to stock lakes in the immediate area as well as throughout the state of Minnesota. Today the ponds are used as interpretive education sites and as resting areas for the region's flocks of migrating waterfowl.

The half-mile trail network is a big loop around the ponds in the complex.

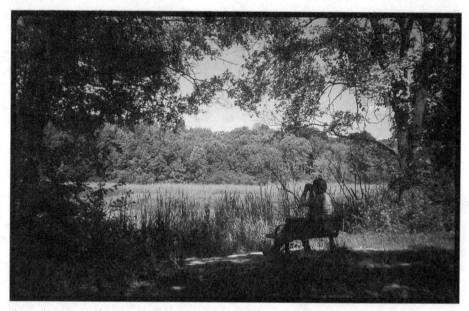

The author pauses for some bird-watching on a bench along the Old Cedar Avenue Trail.

Called the Caretaker's Walk, it offers information on each of the various-sized ponds that collectively are called the Bass Ponds. A descriptive interpretive brochure available at the kiosk is a helpful tool when walking through the history of each pond.

This loop will also put you right at the start of the 1.25-mile trail southwest to Old Cedar Avenue (see Old Cedar Avenue Trail, page 156).

Begin at the information kiosk and take a left along the interpretive trail to the first of 11 sites along the trail (as shown on the refuge map).

Remnants of the original operation are visible at the first two stops. The stairs and decaying foundation of the first clubhouse can be seen as soon as you begin the trail. Continuing on, to the left is Minnow Pond. The pill box structure was used to control the flow and level of water in the ponds. Upstream from this pond was the home of the area's native brook trout. Cold spring water helped them grow 6- to 10-inches in length while living in the creek.

Another one hundred feet and you will come to the Wood Duck Pond. Several wood duck nests were put up in this area. The scientific name of such areas is a "green tree reservoir." Water collects in such depressions long enough for puddle ducks to stop by during migration and feed on seeds and plants on the bottom. Once migration is over and summer follows, these reservoirs dry up, allowing the trees to keep growing. If they remained full of water, many of the trees would drown.

As you continue down the trail, you begin following the shore of Big Bass Pond on your right. Imagine a crew of laborers digging this pond by hand and carting off the excess dirt in wheelbarrows! That's how this was built back in the late 1930s as part of the Work Projects Administration (WPA). Black crappie were raised here.

The spot between the pond and Long Meadow Lake was a jumping-off point for duck hunters seeking flocks of game birds using this area of the lake. Also, there was a commercial fishery where fishermen used to drop gill nets through cuts in the ice to catch carp for a cannery.

Heading southwest, the trail crosses a bridge over the creek from Minnow Pond and continues on past Little Bass Pond's southern bank. Because willow trees root fast and love lots of water and wet soil, they were planted along these ponds so their roots could be used to secure the embankments of the ponds.

Just past this pond is the intersection with a main trail that can take you back to the information kiosk. This is also the trailhead for the 1.25 mile out-and-back trail down to the Old Cedar Avenue Bridge. The next quarter mile continues along the ponds. In the winter, the large pond, called Hog Back Ridge Pond, doesn't always freeze over. Scores of Canada geese and various winter ducks can be seen here.

The trail along Long Meadow Lake continues for about a mile and traces the edge of the lake. Towering cottonwoods and other lowland trees flank the banks for most of its length. This is an incredible birding area. In fact, the entire Minnesota Valley is one of the best corridors in the state for viewing all sorts of birds, both residents and transient migrators. Great blue herons, egrets, puddle ducks, swamp sparrows, red-winged and yellow-headed blackbirds are among literally hundreds of bird species that can be seen along Long Meadow Lake's shoreline. Be sure to bring your spotting scope or binoculars.

Once you pass under Minnesota Highway 77 (Cedar Avenue), you enter marshlands and eventually come upon a few smaller ponds on each side of the road. The terminus of the Bass Pond Trail is at Old Cedar Avenue. The trail comes out just across from the parking lot, the trailhead for the Cedar Trail and the old steel-frame bridge that once carried traffic south along Old Cedar Avenue.

At this point you have several choices: continue on the Old Cedar Avenue trail network; retrace your steps back to the Bass Pond area; continue along Long Meadow Trail another couple of miles to its western terminus at Interstate 35 W; or get in the shuttle car you placed here before you started your trip. Pick a nice, sunny Minnesota day for your hike and you may have a hard time deciding what to do next.

NEARBY ACTIVITIES

The trail system options for the Minnesota Valley Wildlife Refuge are the first activities that come to mind. At least four other trail systems feed off this trail at the southern terminus and beyond. For a totally different walking experience, try hiking the four levels of the great Mall of America just up the road.

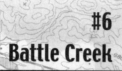

#6
Battle Creek

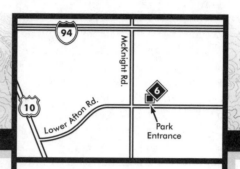

Park
Entrance

IN BRIEF

The southern unit offers the best hiking within this multi-unit park. Mature stands of hardwoods, small ponds nestled in among the trees, and winding, paved paths that dip and climb gently through woods and meadows offer hikers a pleasant, woodsy setting right in the heart of southwest St. Paul.

DIRECTIONS

Head east on Interstate 94, through St. Paul, to McKnight Road, turn right (south) toward Lower Afton Road. Turn left (east) on Lower Afton Road, at 200 yards you'll come to the entrance to parking lot on the left.

DESCRIPTION

There are three distinct units to Battle Creek Park: the northern unit is comprised of a picnic area, playgrounds, and other developed amenities centered around a small lake, the western unit is a trailhead at the end of the ravine through which Battle Creek flows, and the southern unit is a spaghetti network of trails through mature oaks and around marshy lowlands—and the source of our hike of choice.

Begin at the parking lot off of Lower Afton Road. At the far end of the lot is a trailhead for the Pet Trail on the left and a trailhead sign for the bike/hike trail that parallels the parking lot. The sign shows the trails, but the information is

KEY AT-A-GLANCE
INFORMATION

Length: 4.4 miles

Configuration: Irregular circle

Difficulty: Mostly easy walking with some gradual slopes

Scenery: Impressive considering its city location; broad meadows and mature forests

Exposure: Mixture of sun and shade

Traffic: Lots of bike riders and hikers on evenings and weekends

Trail Surface: Paved throughout

Hiking Time: 1½–2 hours

Season: All seasons; some segments are designated ski trails in winter or serve as corridors to many spurs off main route

Access: No fees

Maps: None; trailside map is slightly confusing; stay on paved bike/hike path

Special Comments: Lots of birds, a large variety of trees for a city park

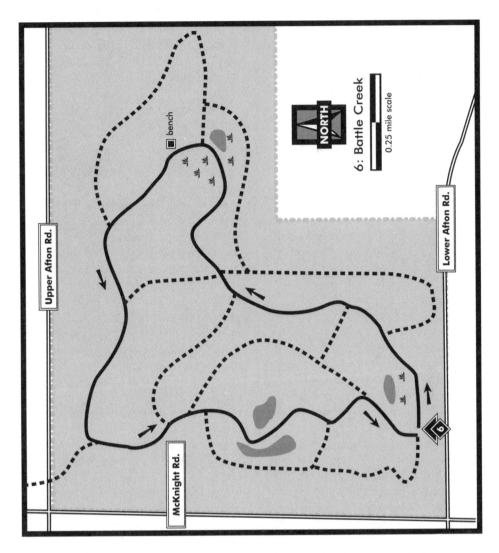

more confusing then helpful. There are no maps printed for Battle Creek of a scale or in sufficient detail to do any good, so the simple rule for this hike is to stay on the paved trail. There is only one intersection where this is challenged. Therefore, a second rule— always take the paved trail to the left—will keep the directions simple for this hike.

Head uphill on the paved trail to the right of the bike/hike sign to begin the hike. As you start up the hill, you pass through typical upland forest species:

oaks and ash, a few scattered pine trees, and a modest understory of saplings and ground vegetation. These trails constantly meander around and through the woods, rising and dipping on a route that follows the rolling contours of the park.

The trail turns to the left into a denser stand of trees. A grass trail to the right is one of many you will encounter along this route—if you do happen upon a map, many of these are not marked, or are marked incorrectly. However, these are all ski trails and as such are grass, not paved.

An adventurous hiker can choose to add these at will and basically create additional loops to expand the hike. All eventually lead back to the main paved trail loop.

Continue on the paved section, past another grassy trail on the left, and through a more mature stand of stately oaks. The trail will continue to meander and rise to an intersection of several trails. One is a utility corridor along a row of pine trees. No matter, stay on the paved trail past this intersection and follow the main trail to the left. Immediately past this intersection, circle around the bottom edge of a huge meadow covered in tall grass and wildflowers.

The trail skirts the southern edge of the meadow then cuts to the right, through the middle of the expansive rolling meadow and down into a small stand of trees—mostly box elders. Trails will approach from both the right and the left but keep the rule in mind and the paved pathway will lead you right down through the islands of trees and along a marshy area on the left.

You are now at the eastern end of the meadow, and the woods rise to your right as the path swings back to the left (north) and around this marshy area. Just before you come to another paved pathway on your right, you'll pass a small pond on the right. This is a good bird-viewing area (the entire park has lots of birds) for ducks and egrets and possibly a great blue heron.

The intersection offers a paved path to the right heading over the crest of the meadow's edge. Stick to the path straight ahead (the left fork) and continue on around the marsh rushes and grasses. About 100 yards along this open section of the trail you'll come to a bench flanked by two huge cottonwoods—giants by any standard—towering over the trail. They are magnificent specimens of what a healthy cottonwood can attain in form and beauty.

The trail enters the woods again as it ascends and descends with the rolling terrain. You will wind through a stand of hardwoods before coming out at another main intersection. This is actually a northern trailhead for this section of the park and is adjacent to the tennis courts. A couple of paved paths lead off to the right at this point but it's clear that you want to stay on the left-most trail to head back into the wooded area. There is a trailhead sign with trails designated, but, like the sign at the southern end, its information is not very clear. From here to the end of the trail, the paved section is the main route and continues to be easy to follow.

The trail dips and turns in a series of S turns through a lowland section of the park for the next mile. You will cross two major intersections, both grass, before winding through a bog area comprised of a couple of small ponds—one on either side of the trail. The path cuts sharply to the left and then sharply to the right as it swings and dips past these two wet areas.

You emerge into an open understory beneath tall maples and box elders before the path rises again as it goes into the final upland wooded area. Another small pond on the left marks the end of the trail as the path opens onto the clearing at the start of the trailhead at the end of the parking lot.

NEARBY ACTIVITIES

Hike through the western section of Battle Creek up a steep, rocky ravine and then through the forested area on the bluffs. This is an out-and-back trail. Park at the Point Douglas Street parking lot just off of US 61.

The Indian Mounds Park 2 miles to the west offers short trails and native history. This park is just north of the Cottage Ravine Trail on US 61.

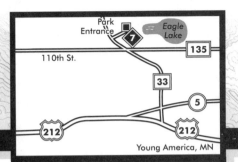

Young America, MN

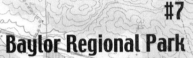

#7
Baylor Regional Park

IN BRIEF

This is a quaint, county-like park with a refreshing maple forest, marsh area, and modestly developed lakefront area. Whether you come to camp and hike or just make it a pleasant afternoon, Baylor offers a peaceful setting.

DIRECTIONS

Head west from Minneapolis on Crosstown 62 or Interstate 494 to the intersection with US Highway 212. Take US 212 west to Minnesota Highway 5. Take MN 5 west about 25 miles to Norwood, Minnesota. In Norwood, take County Road 33 north 2.5 miles to park entrance on the right.

DESCRIPTION

The first impression one gets from entering Baylor Regional Park is that it's not really a park at all but a restored farm site. The large barn right across the parking lot that serves as the park's headquarters and the adjacent caretaker's residence seems reminiscent of a typical midwestern homestead farm in Carver County.

The trail system meanders through nearly all of the park's 230 acres, providing hikers with great views of the lake, walks through thick maple stands, and a floating walkway across a marsh.

From the parking lot alongside the barn, walk between the two main buildings and head toward the campground. Utility camping will be on your left, but

KEY AT-A-GLANCE
INFORMATION

Length: 4.6 miles

Configuration: Three loops off a main trailhead road

Difficulty: Gently rolling and winding trails with gradual and modest rises in sections

Scenery: Young maple forest with some larger trees, expansive marsh area adjacent to a shallow prairie lake

Exposure: Cool shade under the maples, exposed trails near the lake

Traffic: Expect moderate RV-camper use in summer, locals on weekends at picnic area and lake

Trail Surface: Some packed gravel in campground area, compacted earth otherwise

Hiking Time: 1¼–2 hours at a casual pace

Season: All year

Access: $3 daily vehicle fee; $16 annual vehicle fee (only $9.60 annual fee if you have a Hennepin Parks Annual Permit)

Maps: Available at the barn headquarters

Special Comments: Likely to see a variety of migrating waterfowl in spring and summer at marsh and lake areas of park

23

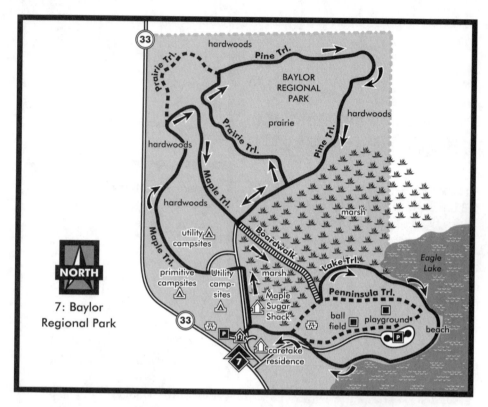

NORTH

7: Baylor
Regional Park

keep going to the first gravel road intersection. This is the start of Maple Trail.
Take a left here and walk past the second
campsite—it's on your right—and head
into the woods just past the bathhouse.

You will quickly see why its called the
"maple" trail. While not big, the maples
are certainly plentiful. These are sugar
maples; you can tell by the rounded
inner corner of the lobes on the leaf (on
red maples this corner forms a right
angle). The trail follows fairly close to
the highway as it heads north. At about
0.2 mile, it swings slightly west toward
the highway but cuts back into more
hardwoods, where older maples dominate. The path passes through a corridor
of arched maple canopies to form a cool,
shaded pathway.

At about a half mile down the Maple
Trail, you will come to an intersection
on your right. This is the continuation of

the Maple back to the camping area. It is
also a way to link up with the other
major loop in this part of the park, so
hang a right and enjoy more young and
mature maples as the trail dips and
curves through more sugar maples.

At the end of the Maple Trail, you will
come out facing the marsh. You are now
at the northern end of the campground
road. Look for the Pine Trail on your
immediate left and take it. You will
return on this section of the Pine Trail
later. For now, follow the path as it skirts
the marsh on your right for about 0.2
mile before you reach another fork. Take
the left fork.

The trail at this point is called the
Prairie Trail, and it cuts back into the
woods. There are more wet areas in this
section since elevations are lower. You will
see a small pond. There is also a dense
stand of mature maples in this section.

You will have traveled about 0.4 mile when the trail forms a T with the Pine Trail. Turn left and you will return to the Maple Trail, but you want to turn right through more hardwoods (maples) and red pines as the trail meanders across the northernmost section of the park. There are some open grassy areas on the right, and the larger marsh at the north end of Eagle Lake is on the left as the trail loops back to where it connects with the Prairie Trail again.

By this point you have taken two loops that have trailed through the wooded area of the park's western and northern reaches. As you meet up with the main trail you will return to the end of the campground road where the trail forked earlier. If you backtrack past the campground on your right you will come to a short spur on the left, right across the road from the first Maple Trail intersection. This spur leads to a boardwalk that crosses the marsh north of Eagle Lake.

The walkway is a floating trail that cuts across the western third of the marsh, putting the hiker a few feet above the water for a short 0.2-mile stretch.

You can also walk the shoreline along the cattails and rushes for a good opportunity to enjoy the marsh from a close (but dry) vantage point.

The end of the boardwalk intersects with the Peninsula Trail to the right and the Lake Trail to the left. The Peninsula Trail loops through a developed recreational area of the park (playground, ball diamond, etc.) while the Lake Trail follows the shoreline of Eagle Lake for about 0.9 mile. Follow the Lake Trail.

For the first quarter mile, the marsh dominates the left side of the trail. Once you come upon the open water of Eagle Lake you'll be able to look out over this body of water for the next 0.4 mile or so. The trail will cut away from the lake and cross the road near the volleyball nets as it heads back toward the park's headquarters. It meets up with the main campground road right behind the caretaker's house across from the headquarters barn.

Nearby Activities
There's a lot to do at this quaint park. After hiking, you can enjoy a picnic or play a game of tennis or volleyball.

#8
Bryant Lake
Figure Eight

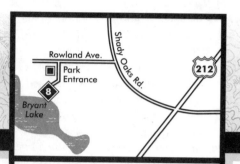

IN BRIEF

Noted for its steep, rolling hills, the park's still-developing trails will ultimately enable hikers to combine a walking workout with glimpses of nature's handiwork preserved in a bustling urban setting.

DIRECTIONS

Head west on Crosstown 62 to the intersection with US Highway 212. Take US 212 west about 0.7 mile to Shady Oak Road/County Road 61. Turn north/right and go 0.3 mile to Rowland Avenue. Turn left and go about one block, then turn left into the park at the sign.

DESCRIPTION

Surrounded by freeways, townhouses, and more highways, the Bryant Lake Trail is a modest route that makes the most of this small, 170+ acre urban park. By capitalizing on every twist and turn within the park, the trail serves two purposes: one as a vigorous workout/power-walking loop; the other as a chance to relax and enjoy terrain and trees more common to rural parks. By combining both walking environments, you'll find that Bryant Lake offers a full-featured, albeit short, figure-eight double loop through the marshy reaches at the area's eastern end.

Start at the parking lots adjacent to the visitor center overlooking Bryant Lake. This is the center of the recreation area and both major hiking paths lead

KEY AT-A-GLANCE INFORMATION

Length: 1.3 miles

Configuration: A very irregular, amoebae-like figure eight

Difficulty: Undulating, with some slippery sections

Scenery: Oak savanna at higher elevations with developing topography from steep slopes

Exposure: Mostly full sun, marshy area in shade

Traffic: Some along the marshy interior—deer take refuge there

Trail Surface: Paved walkways

Hiking Time: 45–60 minutes

Season: Three seasons

Access: $5 daily vehicle permit, $27 Patrons Annual Hennepin Parks permit

Maps: Available at park headquarters or at www.hennepinparks.org

Facilities: Fully developed with picnic area, visitor center, rest rooms, water

Special Comments: Plenty of parking—a nice short hike for busy people

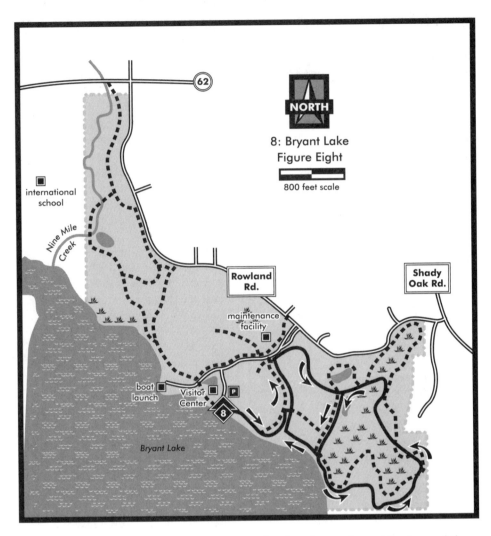

8: Bryant Lake
Figure Eight

800 feet scale

away, east and west, from this central hub. Much of the trail was still under construction when I hiked this park, so many surfaces that were woodchips or bare earth may be paved now.

Head down to the beach and take a left by the bathhouse area to access the shared bike/hike trail which leads into the wooded and wilder eastern section of the park. The trail lies right alongside the lake and the undulating pathway hints at the hilly nature of this small park.

You will soon come to an intersection, take a left and head toward the developed area, the parking lot, and the road into the park. You might as well concentrate on your aerobic breathing, as the scenery is all groomed playground.

As you climb the hill toward the entrance to the park, the trail will swing east and continue to follow the outside perimeter of the most developed area. Continue on beyond this intersection for about 0.2 mile until you intersect with one of the proposed paved trails. Eventually this trail will cut a longer, paved section around the marsh area ahead.

As you reach the trail crossing, you are at the top of the waist on the figure eight. Turn right and continue along the western edge of the marsh area. There is a small pond on your left as soon as you start heading south along this section.

The steep, rolling hills are considered the most striking feature of this park. At the highest point in the park you will be almost 150 feet above the surface of the lake. Some of the slopes are quite steep. Between these extremely steep sides are valley-like chutes, called "swales," that vary in width and all lead back down to the lake. The hills on this trail enable one to launch a power hike along the slopes.

In this section there are two trail intersections that will lead back to the parking lot. However, if you continue on, you'll come to a foot/bike bridge over a small creek.

The trail follows the lake after you pass the second of the two intersections. Then it swings inland along the southern edge of the marshland. The wooded areas are dominated by mature hardwoods (oak, maple) along the southern and central areas. Lower down the slopes toward the lake, the trees and understory vegetation are typical of floodplain flora found throughout this area, such as cottonwoods and ash. This is in sharp contrast to the savanna-like burr oak, hawthorn, and red cedar found higher up in the central and western part of the park.

About 1600 feet after crossing the foot bridge there is another junction in the trail. It may be visible just as both trails turn northwest after heading north for a few hundred yards. This is a trail that leads to a park road that, in turn, connects with a spur off of Shady Oaks Road. It's better to stay on either of the marsh trails and complete the loop along the marsh corridor.

The turf trail turns to the west 800 feet past the intersection with the road. It cuts through the marsh area in two places before completing this half of the figure eight loop. If you have the option (that is, if this new paved section is complete) take the longer, paved trail. There may be a conspicuous fork in the trial leading to the northernmost marshy arm in the park. This trail loops around the arm and returns to the main trail along the top of the figure eight. If this is confusing, just remember you are on a sideways figure eight, the left half is developed, the right half is wooded and marshy. The "waist" of the figure eight splits the two sections north-to-south.

Be on the watch for deer. At dusk, in October, I witnessed four deer entering this wild area from the backyards of the condos to the north and east. Again, for such a small park, its amenities are impressive.

Once you reach the western edge of the marsh you are back at the upper end of the waist on the figure eight. Head south again. There will be marsh on one side and a steep slope on the other. At the other end of this section you will come to a T intersection. Take the trail back along the lake and toward the parking lot.

NEARBY ACTIVITIES

The park has a modern visitor center, boat launch, and fishing pier. Another proposed trail network will provide a small loop trail to the west of the visitor center. Northwestern Trail along Nine Mile Creek leads out of the park and connects with trails from Eden Prairie and Minnetonka.

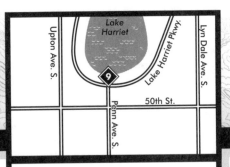

IN BRIEF

This hike is a section of the Grand Round Parkway Trail System, passing around Minneapolis's two largest lakes, visiting another intimate lake for bird watching, and taking an optional side trip to a culturally diverse neighborhood.

DIRECTIONS

From 50th Street and Lyndale Avenue South in Minneapolis, head west on 50th Street to Penn Avenue. Turn north and go about 2 blocks to 48th Street and Lake Harriet Parkway. Parking spaces can be found along the many turn-outs along the parkway. There is additional parking on most side streets.

DESCRIPTION

Like most parkway trail systems, the City Lakes Chain can be entered or exited anywhere along the pathway. You can also link this hike with several other hikes found elsewhere in the book, including the Lake Nokomis, Minneha-ha Falls, and Mississippi Gorge hikes.

While going around the lakes, the Parks and Recreation Board requests that people walk in a clockwise direction to help maintain an efficient and safe pedestrian traffic flow. With this in mind, begin the trail at the extreme south end of the lake (where Penn Avenue meets Lake Harriet Parkway at about 48th Street) and head to the left (clockwise). This is an area of small vegetation and willow

KEY AT-A-GLANCE INFORMATION

Length: 10.8 miles, full loop

Configuration: Three stacked loops with connecting spurs

Difficulty: Completely flat except for the William Berry Parkway, which is a 0.5-mile uphill climb

Scenery: City park, with stunning skyline views of Minneapolis from the south shore of each lake

Exposure: Mostly full sun; some shade along lakes and corridors

Traffic: Very popular throughout summer, but never seems crowded

Trail Surface: Paved throughout; pedestrian-only pathways for most of route

Hiking Time: 5–6½ hours (about 2 hours for each lake)

Season: All year

Access: No fees

Maps: Available from Minneapolis Parks and Recreation (ask for The Grand Rounds Parkway System); also check city maps of Minneapolis with good detail of the lakes

Facilities: Rest rooms, drinking water, concession stands at main beach of each lake

Special Comments: For exercise or leisure, these trails are among the best in Minneapolis, and lit at night

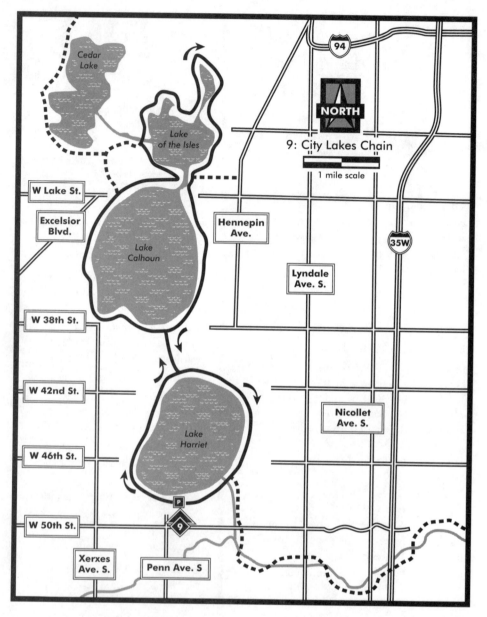

1 mile scale

clumps along the shoreline. The area on the other side of the path is mostly spacious and open. Landscaped sections and fishing docks add a rustic touch to the setting. A wooden, arched footbridge just before a section called Beard's Plaisante (on a knoll overlooking the lake) completes the rustic, country atmosphere of this section of the lake.

The parkway is a narrow road along the west side of the lake bordering an embankment thick with buckthorns, cherry, and a variety of landscape shrubbery. You'll notice that all the recreational development has been concentrated in the northwest section of Lake Harriet, about 1.2 miles into the hike. The mooring area for small sailboats, the concession stand, and Lake Harriet's most famous landmark—the band shell—can be found here. Summer concerts at Lake Harriet draw audiences from the city and beyond. A great way to relax during a hike is to sit and listen to the wide assortment of musical programs available here. Some people will rent or bring canoes and listen from just off shore.

If you are continuing around the chain, you will now head to the left through the parking area, past the picnic area, and along William Berry Parkway. This pathway winds about 0.5 mile through a woodland of mature oaks and maples running parallel to the parkway toward the south end of Lake Calhoun (the equivalent of about 38th Street South and Russell Avenue).

Lake Calhoun is big and round, actually very typical of those lakes throughout Minnesota that were formed when massive blocks of ice gouged a basin out of the old seabed or earlier glacial deposits. Upon melting, they left depressions filled with water to become lakes. The path follows this lake right along the shoreline for its entire length. Stately elms and hackberries provide shade over the expansive lawns. It's mostly open air with wide, grassy play areas for much of the 3.1-mile walk around Calhoun.

Again traveling clockwise, the trail soon passes an area known as Thomas Beach—it has gone through many cultural phases but continues to be a hang out spot because of the beach and its sand volleyball courts.

At the northwest end of Calhoun looms the stately Calhoun Beach Hotel, a neighborhood landmark for years. There is a parkway route alongside the hotel that connects with the Cedar Lake Parkway, which bypasses the Lake of the Isles area. To make use of the full scope of the chain, however, stay to the right along the north shore. You will pass the large swimming area, beach, and parking area and continue on toward the concession stand and mooring area at the northeast corner of Calhoun. If you intend to walk to Lake of the Isles, you may want to drop down to the right and freshen up at the concession stand. There are no facilities at Lake of the Isles.

Head back north across West Lake Street and up Dean Parkway toward Lake of the Isles. The path actually follows a channel between the two lakes, under one bridge and along a built-up side of the channel. The path is 0.6-mile long and goes under a second bridge before opening out onto Lake of the Isles Parkway at its most southern end.

Lake of the Isles is probably the shallowest of the lakes, and at low water it can be less than appealing. However, the serpentine trail winds around two arms of the lake on the northern half, giving the hike a little more character than the two circular routes of the southern lakes.

The southwestern section of the trail is a bit more hilly than the trails of the other lakes. As the trail curves around to the west side, a footbridge comes into view. This passes over another channel that connects Lake of the Isles to Cedar Lake. Again, this is an opportunity to continue on the grand tour and head west to the trail around the west end of Cedar Lake and points north. However, to fulfill the Lake Chain, you should continue on over the bridge to the north.

As the trail cuts through this section, the trees come closer to the lake, thereby providing a little shade. The trail soon swings right and down to the water's edge where a built-up bank keeps the trail from falling off into the water.

This is also the point on the lake route that brings you closest to the two islands situated in the center of the lake. Both islands are small, isolated reserves. If you are a birder, or just curious about nature, bring binoculars. Frequently, there is at least one of several wetland bird species roosting along the shore or in the trees. I've seen green herons, great blue herons, and egrets along these shores.

The northeasternmost part of the lake is a narrow finger that sticks up into the Kenwood district. A neighborhood park with tennis courts and playgrounds is nearby. From here the trail follows the east side of the lake.

At this point you have completed nearly 5 miles of the Lake Loop. If you want to shorten your hike into a one-way hike, this would be a good place to park a shuttle vehicle, since there is plenty of street parking along the parkway and side streets. However, persevere if you can because the entire eastern shoreline of the lakes awaits you.

When you reach the south end of Lake of the Isles you can double back along the channel or, if you want to enjoy a little neighborhood walking, exit the parkway. Head east along Lake Street to the heart of the Lake and Hennipen districts where you'll find gift shops, ethnic restaurants, and places to rent bicycles and inline skates.

After you have had your fill of restaurants and shopping, return to the hike by heading west along West Lake Street to Lake Calhoun. There is a flower garden and a flagpole marking the head of the lake. There used to be a gigantic river boat pilot house wheel at the base of the flag pole but it was stolen many years ago. Head for the concession stand and continue along the pathway to the left that parallels the dense stand of trees and shrubs.

About 0.75 mile south of the concession stand area you will come to the intersection with William Berry Parkway. Take this 0.56-mile climb up to the

parkway around Lake Harriet, where it intersects with the concession stand/ bandstand area of the lake.

Walk east here (left) and past the swimming beach. This section of the beach has a windswept feel to it, several of the pine trees have that Monterey Bay look to them. As the trail turns to follow the lake to the south, you can make another side trip to the Rose Garden and bird sanctuary. Well-manicured beds of roses are showcased here. Naturally, from late spring through summer you'll find the roses in full bloom.

This last section of Lake Harriet offers a peaceful promenade close to the shoreline with many spots to drop down into the water to cool tired feet. About 0.7 mile past the rose garden, at about West 46th Street, there is a small swimming beach that is very popular among families with small children. It's also a major intersection with the bike trail, the pedestrian trail, and serves as an entrance to the lake paths from the parkway and adjoining city streets.

At this point the path is routed through a canopy of branches that form a tunnel for several hundred feet. Gnarly oaks, maples, buckthorns, and willows are the dominant species in this area. Just beyond this cool, shaded tunnel is another open space—and the wooden bridge where the loop started nearly 10 miles earlier.

Nearby Activities

The Hennepin-Lake area just east of Lake Calhoun is one of Minneapolis's most visited street corners. Specialty shops, great ethnic restaurants, and scores of handmade crafts create a mini cultural area. You can even rent bicycles and in-line skates to use around the lakes.

#10
Cleary Lake
Regional Park

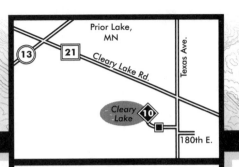

IN BRIEF

A moderately long hike around a pleasant lakeside setting. Nothing fancy here in the way of natural amenities, but has that "walk in the park" feel to it. A good hiking trail for a relaxed gait or for an aerobic workout.

DIRECTIONS

Located southeast of Prior Lake. Take Minnesota Highway 13 to Eagle Creek Parkway (County Road 21), then to Texas Avenue (CR 27). Head south to park entrance. Access from Interstate 35W south to Lakeville. Go west on Cleary Lake Road (CR 21) through Keatings to Texas Avenue (CR 27) and north to the park entrance. Turn left and drive to the main parking area at end of road.

DESCRIPTION

This is one of those casual hiking areas where you can amble along at a slow pace or speed walk for some aerobic exercise. The 3.8-mile trail encircles the lake along a gradually undulating pathway that hikers of all levels can enjoy.

The lake covers over 137 acres of the northern half of the park. Geographically, the park is situated in ground moraine, deposited during the last Ice Age—specifically the Superior and Des Moines lobes. It's one of the area's bigger parks—covering over 1,100 acres—and much of it is still undeveloped.

KEY AT-A-GLANCE INFORMATION

Length: 3.8 miles

Configuration: A basic loop following the lake's shoreline

Difficulty: Very easy, mostly level, with gradual rises and gentle dips

Scenery: Open country, suburban setting on periphery, views of lake

Exposure: Trail is 80% open, hot on intensely sunny days

Solitude: Fairly well used, but room for everyone at their own pace

Trail Surface: 8-feet wide, bituminous surface with a center line

Hiking Time: 1½–2 hours at a casual pace

Season: All seasons; separate ski trails in winter

Access: $5 daily vehicle permit, $27 Patrons Annual Hennepin Parks permit

Maps: Available at park headquarters or www.hennepinparks.org

Facilities: Drinking water, playground, boat launch, rest rooms, picnic area, nearby golf course and clubhouse

Special Comments: If a "walk around the lake" is your kind of hike, Cleary Lake is your kind of lake

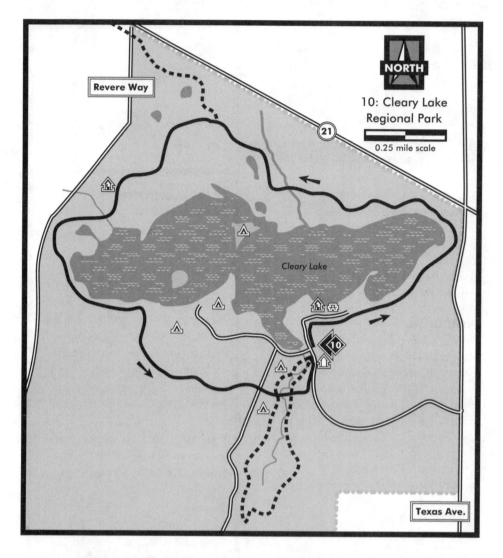

10: Cleary Lake
Regional Park

0.25 mile scale

Revere Way

21

Cleary Lake

10

Texas Ave.

There are about 6 miles of ski trails throughout the southern half of the park. However, for summer hiking the route around Cleary Lake is the relaxing way to go.

Starting at the parking lot, follow the wide, paved hike/bike trail north and to the right around the southeastern portion of the lake. A small finger of land, a hooked peninsula, juts out from the shoreline right past the end of the parking area. The bays you pass feature aquatic vegetation common to lakes in this area.

The trail rises to a ridge and then levels off as it continues around the east end of the lake. Most of this area has islands of trees, albeit none at a mature height. Spruce trees beyond a shoulder fringe of grasses line the trail paralleling the golf course.

As the trail turns westward along the northern shoreline a trail junction marks the intersection of a proposed regional trail connection. Ultimately, this park will be linked with a trail system connecting Murphy-Hanrehan Regional

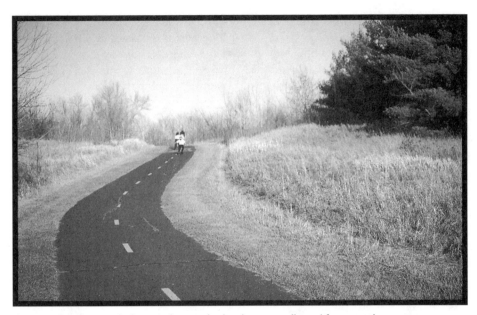

The paved trail around Cleary Lake suits both relaxing strolls and fast-paced exercise.

Park. The northeast corner of Cleary is only 1 mile west of the southwest corner of its regional park neighbor. This section of the trail will also be part of a longer, multi-park corridor to the west.

County Road 21 forms the northern boundary of the park and the trail continues along its meandering route over gently rolling hills (very modest changes in grade). About half a mile along this segment, the trail crosses a small creek. There is a marsh area on the left. Just past this creek the trail follows the proposed boundary of one of the recreation areas that will be developed as part of the park's master plan. It will include more picnic areas, a launch facility for non-motorized boats, and another swimming area. This section of the park also contains several smaller ponds in a wetlands section at the north end of the lake.

About 1200 feet past the creek there is yet another trail intersection. This is a junction with the Scott County West Regional Trail. Once completed and linked, these trails (Scott, Cleary Lake,

and Murphy-Hanrehan) will stretch from just west of I-35W south to Prior Lake.

The trail now follows the northwest shoreline as it winds southward. This part of the park is open country and is a bit higher in elevation than the eastern side. The path parallels County Road 87 for nearly two-thirds of a mile. It crosses another creek and loops around a small bay at the extreme western end of Cleary Lake. There is a small island in this bay. Eventually, this last section plus about a quarter of the southern perimeter of the lake will be skirted by a park road that will follow alongside this hike/bike trail. For now, however, its a peaceful route through rolling, open grassland areas.

After crossing over yet another creek, this one flowing out of the extreme southwestern point of the lake's shoreline, the trail continues for about another 1400 feet before it turns sharply to the south and away from the lake. It cuts through stands of spruce and weaves its way toward the west central portions of the park. Here a large woodland of oak and aspen dominates the scene. There are 4.4 miles of cross-country ski trails in the southern half of the park. One of the main access trails to this network crosses the hiking path at about 0.2 mile from the point where the trail turns away from the lake.

The trail continues for about a third of a mile before coming to the main park road. It's another quarter mile back to the main parking area. The trail comes up to the lake just east of the 125-foot-long swimming beach. A dip in Cleary Lake can be a cool way to end one's hike—on a hot day this black, paved pathway is going to bake!

NEARBY ACTIVITIES

Murphy-Hanrehan Regional Park is situated just 1 mile to the east. Prior Lake, Savage, and Shakopee all offer myriad activities.

#11
Clifton E. French
Regional Park

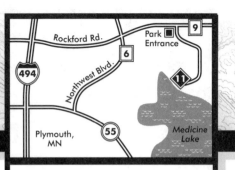

IN BRIEF

What was merely an underutilized marshy area surrounded by cone-shaped mounds of glacial gravel has been developed into one of the most activities-diverse parks in the Regional Parks system. Hikers may want to bring a fishing pole and swimsuit along with their hiking shoes.

DIRECTION

Drive west from Minneapolis on Minnesota Highway 55/Olsen Memorial Highway to Medicine Lake Drive. Go right (north) onto Northwest Boulevard (County Road 61) for about three quarters of a mile to Rockford Road (CR 9). Turn right/east and travel for about 0.25 mile to the park entrance. Follow the winding, hilly roadway to the far parking lot. The trail begins at the shuttle stop near the complex that includes the boat rental area, boat launch, and swimming beach.

DESCRIPTION

Like several other urban Minneapolis parks, Clifton E. French Regional Park is completely surrounded by concrete corridors and building complexes. Still, it preserves a glimpse of what this country around the northern shores of Medicine Lake looked like long before development took a foothold.

When driving into the park, one senses the scope of Clifton E. French Park.

KEY AT-A-GLANCE INFORMATION

Length: 1.75 miles

Configuration: Barbell

Difficulty: Rolling pathway with some steep inclines; paved around marshes, beach, and boat launch

Scenery: Pleasantly woodsy with rolling hills, southern exposure to lake and marsh country

Exposure: Mostly full sun, some shade

Traffic: Promoted as a multi-use park, lots of activities all year long

Trail Surface: 1-mile loop is paved; wooded arm is packed turf

Hiking Time: 1 hour

Season: All seasons; especially busy in winter due to lit ski trails

Access: $5 daily vehicle permit, $27 Patrons Annual Hennepin Parks permit

Maps: Available at park headquarters or at www.hennepinparks.org

Facilities: Recreation area, visitor center, drinking water, rest rooms, lights, beach, and boat launch

Special Comments: One of several regional corridor trails leads off the 1-mile loop and heads south along US Highway 169 but does not yet connect to another trail

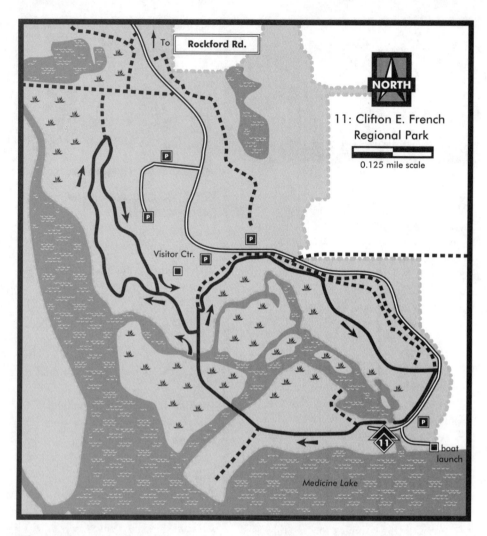

NORTH

11: Clifton E. French
Regional Park

0.125 mile scale

P

P

Visitor Ctr.

P

P

P

11

boat
launch

Medicine Lake

The marshes are in depressions in the kettle moraine left from the most recent glaciation. These depressions are flanked by formations called "kames"—conical hills with steep slopes. Geologically, this is a landscape of mixed Grantsburg and Superior Drift plain. It was formed primarily from till and outwash deposited from massive glaciers. Imagine this entire area before being "leveled" by freeway construction and mega malls. The slopes of some of the narrow-topped ridges and hills along this hike remain quite steep.

There are actually over 10 miles of hiking trails within the park's borders. All of these include at least a view of the park's central attraction, Medicine Lake. There is a shoreline of more than 2 miles, part of which is a 0.75-mile, 38-acre, arm-like bay that stretches north beyond the main body of the lake. Flanked by marshes and steep ridges, the terrain offers hikers changes in elevation and topography completely different from the development that surrounds it.

Like most of the regional parks and some of the state and municipal ones, too, French has designated pet/hike trails—over 4 miles of such pathways. These are basically aligned along the north/south ridge that flanks the western border of the park and provides a buffer between CR 60/Northwest Boulevard and the long arm of the lake. This area includes islands of young aspen and some oaks interspersed among open meadowlands.

With that in mind, I have selected two loops that can be combined into one 1.5-mile hike that includes both a paved trail and a turf pathway.

Follow the shore of the main lake west past the swimming beach. In about 0.3 mile you will come to a road on the left that leads to the picnic area. Keep going over the bridge and over one of the many estuary channels in this area (good birding here, particularly in the extensive marshland to the east). As you continue over a second bridge, you begin to leave the marshy area and enter the steep-ridges topography between the arm of the lake and the visitor center.

After crossing this second bridge, take the turf hiking trail which cuts off to the left. This is the beginning of a 0.75-mile loop through some of the more unique terrain in the park. About 600 feet past the trail junction, you will come to a fork in the path—the high road and low road along the lake's outstretched arm. Take the left fork, which follows the low road. At the northern end of the loop, you'll see a path on the left that provides access to the rest of the park's trails, including the pet walk.

Continue on the upper trail and return through the same wooded area of gnarly oaks and maples. This loop section is actually a few hundred feet shorter, so you'll soon arrive at the southern intersection. Retrace your steps to the paved loop trail you left earlier and turn left.

This paved promenade continues its 1-mile loop around the marsh area and parallels the roadway as it becomes more sidewalk than hiking trail. After meeting the roadway the trail sticks close beside it for another 800 feet before breaking away at an optional fork in the trail that enables hikers to cut back into the marshy area one last time before coming to the boat launch complex.

NEARBY ACTIVITIES

Medicine Lake sees its share of fishing pressure—for presumably good reason. Also, the City of Plymouth's bike/hike trail connects with the park road at the park's entrance and continues west on Rockford Road/CR 90 and then south along Northwest Boulevard/CR 61 for added trekking.

Clifton E. French Park has been developed as one of four official winter recreation parks in the Hennepin Park network. The Hennipen Parks headquarters is located at the north end of the park. This is also a good source of maps and information on the other parks in their system, most of which are featured in this book.

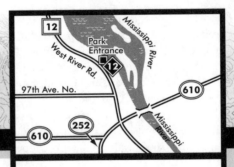

#12
Coon Rapids Dam

IN BRIEF

In addition to the large expanse of concrete across the Mississippi River, Coon Rapids Regional Park offers several miles of trails through lowland/floodplain flora and fauna along the Mississippi's banks. The trail follows the main channel and backwaters of the Mississippi along its course.

DIRECTIONS

From the Twin Cities, take Interstate 94 north past I-694 to Minnesota Highway 252 (MN 252 then becomes MN 610 just before it crosses the river). Turn left (west) onto West River Road and go 0.5 mile to Russell Avenue (MN 12). Turn right (north) on Russell for about 0.75 mile to find the park entrance on the right. Park at the northernmost parking lot or at the ranger station/visitor center.

DESCRIPTION

While the key feature that draws visitors to this park is a restored dam across the Mississippi River, it's the primitive bottomlands along the riverbank that provide the appeal for many hikers.

The trail system includes elongated loops, one on each side of the river. The west bank is less developed, with trails that follow the river and provide close views of the Coon Islands in the channel.

Starting at the parking lot, take the foot path that drops to the river from behind the visitor center. This is a shortcut path

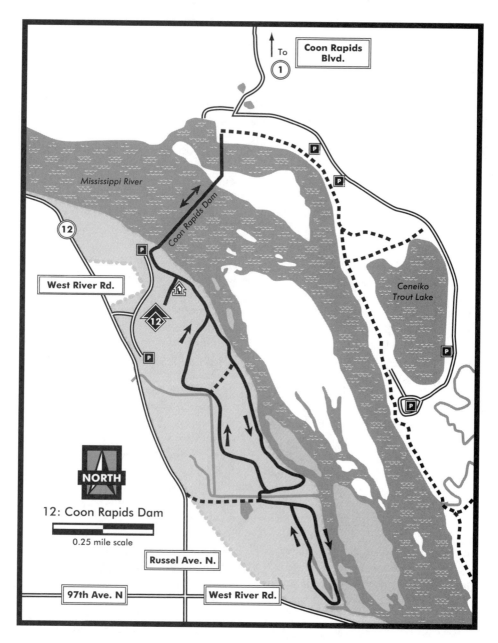

that connects to the river trail at the end of the dam structure. At the intersection with the river, turn right and head downstream.

At about 0.1 mile, you'll see a trail intersection to the right. It is the other end of the big loop that continues through the wooded portion of the west side of the park. Better to stay along the river and follow this path near the water's edge. The view across the river here is unobstructed. Farther on, trees and shrubs along the embankment will make viewing the river channel harder.

After an eigth of a mile, another trail leads to the right. It, too, connects back to the returning loop route. Keep on the main trail. Lowland growth consisting of dogwoods, alders, and box elder dominate the trees in this area. The path is a grassy and earthen trail about four feet wide. There are several thin spots in the growth along the trail's left flank to allow for side trips down to the river.

The trail continues on for another 0.3 mile before turning sharply to the right (west). After another eighth of a mile, you cross a small footbridge over a creek and continue down along the stream's confluence with the Mississippi River.

The trail loops around for another 0.6 miles and meets back up at the bridge again. Hikers can re-trace their route to get glimpses of the river in the opposite direction or head back through the wooded area to the visitor center, about 0.75 mile farther.

This side of the river along the bank is great for bird watching, especially in the spring when floodwaters push the edge of the river way up the banks. The wooded loop section intersects with the riverbank trail about an eighth of a mile from the visitor center, completing loop of about 2.2 miles.

At this point you can follow the pathway north along the river, through a small cut in the vegetation, to the western base of the dam. Here you'll see a small observation deck that enables you to get a crane's-eye view across the entire spillway of the dam. Follow the paved pathway up and around to get on top of the dam for another short hike across the river.

The restored dam uses a portion of the original dam built by Northern States Power (NSP) in 1913 to provide hydroelectric power. Fifty-five years later, in 1968, it was determined that hydropower was no longer efficient, so the dam was phased out of service. Almost 30 years later, a large reconstruction project saw some of the river structures removed along with the top of the dam. This left the walkway that is used today. Although you can't see them, the dam is now controlled by inflatable gates that can be manipulated to control the amount of water flowing through the dam.

It's not quite a quarter mile between the west bank and the path's terminus at Dunn Island. There is another section beyond Dunn Island that connects the dam to the mainland. It provides a water channel enabling boats to bypass the dam. Part of the park's designated amenities include a large pool above the dam for boating and fishing enthusiasts.

You can take this trip across the dam and back (adding about 0.75 mile to your trek) or you can continue on the network of hiking trails laid out along the river on its east bank. The northern sections are slated to have paved walkways and feature stands of oak and a five-acre prairie restoration project.

Turning south after crossing the dam, the trail departs from the visitor center on this side of the river and follows the bank throughout the entire length of the park. There are several stops along the way, including a view of Cenaiko Trout Lake and some of the development just above the lake.

The east bank trail connects with other trails that extend beyond the park and along the river.

NEARBY ACTIVITIES

The North Hennepin Regional Trail extends west from Coon Rapids Dam to Elm Creek Park Reserve.

#13
Cottage Grove
Ravine Regional Park

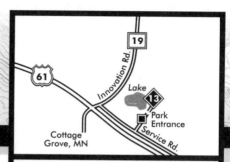

IN BRIEF

Moderate ravine country with solidly wooded slopes and climbs in elevation that reward you with some mid-distance vistas of meadows and farmland "up on top." Trails make it easy to climb and descend from ravine to ridge to ravine throughout the park.

DIRECTIONS

From Minneapolis or southern St. Paul, take Interstate 494 to US Highways 10 and 61 south toward Hastings. Exit at County Road 19 (the exit past 90th Street), go up and over US 61 to the service road heading south. The park entrance is about 0.2 mile on left.

DESCRIPTION

Twenty years ago, I was a county planner in Washington County. Cottage Grove Regional Park was one of my projects for developing the area's recreational potential. At that time the county didn't own as much land as it does now, so development was limited to the overlook parking area and the picnic area at the western edge of the lake. Now, two decades later, I am happy to report that additional land means additional areas for trail development; and what a network of trails it is!

The ravines in this park are quite impressive. Most drain into to the Mississippi about a mile to the west and only a few miles north from where the

KEY AT-A-GLANCE INFORMATION

Length: 2 miles

Configuration: Loop

Difficulty: Moderate with drops and rises through ravines

Scenery: Mature stands of oak, maple, birch, plus steep-sided ravines; lots of great stands of pines in the northern half

Exposure: Mostly full shade below, many open, sunny spaces on top—in the northern half

Traffic: Not too well known, lots of trails for sneaking off

Trail Surface: Packed turf

Hiking Time: 1–1½ hours

Season: All seasons; in winter the major loop is dedicated to cross-country skiing, but other trails are great for hiking or snowshoeing

Access: Washington County Parks fees: $4 daily pass; $20 annual pass; reciprocity with Carver and Anoka County Parks passes

Maps: Available at trailhead near picnic pavilion at far end of northern parking lot

Facilities: Picnic pavilion, rest rooms, drinking water

Special Comments: This area offers a nice balance of ravine climbing and upper-meadow hiking

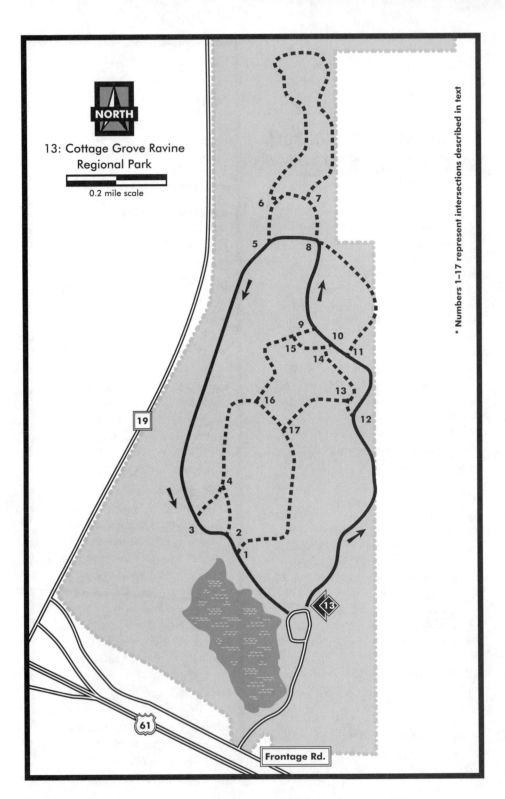

St. Croix joins it on its way south. An interpretive map near the picnic pavilion shows the interconnecting array of trails that have been cut through the ravine and upper meadows. All trail intersections have numbered posts to make map reading virtually foolproof.

From the parking lot, take the far right trail heading north. The path climbs casually but steadily, passing birch, maple, ash, and other old-stand hardwoods that line the ravine feeding southward toward the lake at Cottage Grove. As you approach intersection 12 you'll see more aspen mixed in with the hardwoods.

Continue hiking straight ahead, and just beyond this intersection, after about 80 yards or so, you'll come to an open swath of grass through the woods. This is an underground utilities corridor that bisects the park and continues to its western boundary at CR 19. It's a good reference point when hiking any of the trails along either side of trail intersections 12 and 16.

The trail follows this corridor for about 0.2 mile, leading hikers through upland oaks and a few more aspens. You are above the ravines at this point, and, although wooded, the terrain is more even. Pass intersection 11, one of several options that offer diversity in the park. All side trails tend to join with the main trail after only two- or three-tenths of a mile.

Continue past intersection 10 and reach intersection 9, which appears to be the highest point in the park. From here, the trails to the north tend to wind through wooded or cleared cropland. Continue north along the main trail, leaving the cleared utility corridor behind. The trees here include more oak, some cedar and pines, more aspen, and the understory includes snowberry and sumac. The park then opens up to meadow-like grasslands with islands of

trees throughout. A line of white pines delineates one section of grasslands, while sumac, willows, and ash trees are encroaching other open areas.

Just past the row of pines, more meadow-like areas provide longer vistas of the rolling hills and meadows to the east. Other stands of pines can be seen from this elevated area of the park. This area of Cottage Grove is similar to the neighboring parks to the east that border the St. Croix—high-meadow bluff tops with steep, tree-covered ravines cutting down toward the main drainages.

At intersection 8, turn left and follow a short but steep descent to intersection 5, which quickly brings you into ravine country. The understory is predominantly prickly ash and sumac, and trees typical of lower slopes and ravines again dominate.

Approximately 0.1 mile south of this intersection is the westernmost edge of the same utility corridor you crossed earlier. At this point, you are about 0.5 mile from the northwest tip of the park's main lake. From here the trail descends at a steady, unchanging rate.

Just before the trail turns sharply to the left and the lake comes into view, you'll see a well-worn but unmarked trail to the left. Take this spur trail about 40 yards to a small pond not shown on the map. Look for ducks and more-reclusive shore birds here in the summer—quietly.

Return to the main trail and continue on. As you reach the lake's shore you'll cross intersection 2. If you want to add a 0.5-mile loop to the hike, turn left and keep to the right at all intersections until you come out on the main trail at intersection 1 just 80 yards farther down the trail from intersection 2.

Some maps show a trail completely around the lake in the basin in Cottage Grove Ravine Park. I saw no evidence of the trail around the far side of the lake. I could find no access trail from the extreme northwest end, either. Stick to the north side of the lake for a glimpse of the other shoreline. A good set of binoculars will keep you from missing any scenery or critters.

The trail follows the lake for about 0.2 mile before returning to the parking-and-picnic area.

NEARBY ACTIVITIES

There are several parks and hiking areas along the US 61 corridor, both to the north and south of Cottage Grove Ravine. US 10 leads south to Point Douglas Park at the confluence of the Mississippi and St. Croix rivers. Right across the river is Prescott, Wisconsin.

#14
Crosby Farm Park

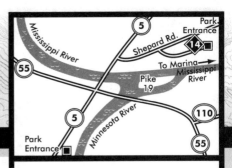

IN BRIEF

Crosby Farm contains a hidden patch of history right at the confluence of the Mississippi and Minnesota rivers. Trails follow the river and wind through the bottomlands and marshes beneath the sheer bluffs near downtown St. Paul.

DIRECTIONS

From Ford Parkway, drive south on Cleveland to Mississippi River Boulevard and then turn left on Shepard Road; park entrances are on the right. The second exit is on the right after another 1.5 miles. From Interstate 35 East in downtown St. Paul, take the Shepard Road exit west to Crosby Road and the eastern park entrance. For the western park entrance, go 1.5 miles past the eastern entrance to the marina sign. Turn left and follow the road past the marina to the entrance and Crosby Farm Museum. From Minnesota Highway 55, go north to MN 5, exit at Shepard Road, and follow the directions above.

DESCRIPTION

There's a lot of history along the Mississippi River, some of it big and bold like Fort Snelling and some barely noticeable beyond the bluff line. Such is the case of Crosby Farm.

When Thomas Crosby and his wife Emma first came to this site on the Mississippi River in 1858, they found an area already bustling with activity. Fort

KEY AT-A-GLANCE INFORMATION

Length: 2.8 miles (side trails and cut throughs add a mile or so more)

Configuration: Elongated figure eight with additional shortcuts and extensions up and down the river

Difficulty: Flat bottomlands, can be slippery when wet and muddy

Scenery: Classic Mississippi River bottomlands with extended and frequent views of the river and Pike Island across the river

Exposure: Mostly shaded with morning sun along riverbank

Traffic: Peaceful, with an undiscovered feeling about it

Trail Surface: Wide, paved walkway with one section of boardwalk

Hiking Time: 1–2 hours

Season: All seasons; great for skiing or snowshoeing in winter

Access: No fees

Maps: Check at Nature Center or www.ci.stpaul.mn.us/depts/parks/

Facilities: Nature center, picnic area, no other development

Special Comments: You literally drop down out of the Twin Cities and into an area that probably looks the same as it did when first farmed more than 150 years ago

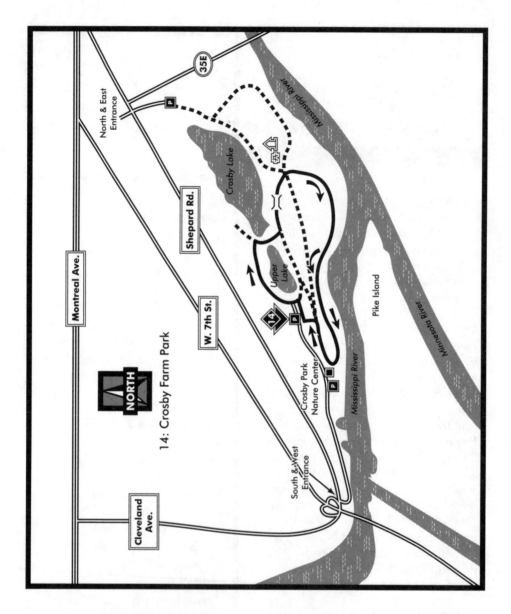

14: Crosby Farm Park

Snelling, completed in 1825 to protect early settlers, loomed on the bluffs above Pike Island. Just downstream, a growing settlement founded by "Pig's Eye" Perrant would eventually become St. Paul. Crosby, an English immigrant, found 160 acres in the floodplain of the Mississippi River, just beyond the point where the Minnesota joins the Mississippi and located just downstream on the Missis-

sippi from Fort Snelling. Today this narrow, 2-mile-long floodplain is Crosby Farm Regional Park. The site of the old Crosby farm is at the southern end of the park, and trails run along the base of the bluff line, across marshy areas, and parallel to the river throughout this slice of river bottomland.

There are two entrances to this park, both off of Shepard Road. This hike

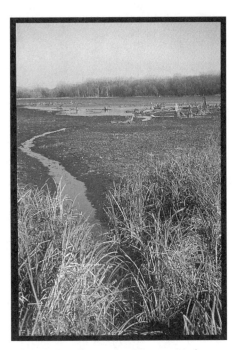

Crosby Lake offers a classic example of Mississippi River bottomlands.

the intersection with the left trail as it loops around Upper Lake. The trail then leads over a footbridge and continues toward the river.

Some 40 yards farther you'll come to a small shelter at the intersection with two other trails. This junction offers you three options. The trail to the left follows the eastern side of Crosby Lake and leads to the north entrance of the park. You can take this out-and-back for an extra mile of hiking. Gigantic cottonwood trees, some over 6 feet in diameter, highlight this trail.

The trail to the right cuts through the center of the park. At the southern end you can either circle back along the river or continue on to the picnic shelter near the park entrance.

However, we'll continue on by going straight through the intersection and continuing on the trail that leads to the river and then swings south, taking you down the riverbank and through the lowlands back to the far southern end of Crosby Park.

The trail follows the curve and contour of the banks of the Mississippi River. Huge cottonwood trees, like sentinels guarding the river, stand along the shoreline. There's not much understory here—it's all been swept away by repeated high waters in the spring. Most of the other trees throughout the area are ash and maple. Sometimes there's a tangle of downed trees and broken limbs, but mostly its an open area with small plants doing their best to be tall on one season's growth.

Since a major flooding in the summer of 2000, this area has been devoid of most understory litter. In its place is a large covering of very fine sand stretching many, many yards back from the river. In the fall, the maple leaves on this barren but sandy forest floor give the area an almost surreal appearance, especially

begins at the westernmost (or southern) entrance. It's the same entrance used for the marina.

Begin at the second parking lot beyond the museum; there the trail heads north through alders and willows to the south end of Upper Lake. Upper and Crosby lakes are nestled close to the base of the bluffs. Fed by the spring floods of the Mississippi, these two lakes are shallow and lined with marsh vegetation along their banks.

The trail forks at Upper Lake: one trail heads to the left and goes between the bluff and the lake, the other goes right along the south edge of the marsh. This loop is an interpretive trail featuring two dozen stations with information on the flora and fauna of the area. For this hike, take the left fork and go around the lake, enjoying the wooden walkway at the northern third of this lake. If you take the right fork, you will soon come to with low autumn sun cutting through the trees.

Occasionally, you will find trails leading off through the floodplain or continuing along the river as the main trail turns inward. These all end up connecting to the main loop—they've been carved out of the understory by years of creative bushwacking.

The trail continues along the river for the full length of the park. As you approach the southern end of the park you can look to the south and practically throw a stone onto Pike Island. Imagine the activity in this area 150 years ago. Today, it's a quiet, casual park hidden below the banks of the river that created it. It's like a mini Fort Snelling Park—only less crowded.

The trail cuts back into the bottomlands, where it intersects with the trail that bisects the park parallel to the river (the second trail choice you had back at the covered shelter). Take a left at the intersection to head to the picnic area or take a right to reconnect with the shelter for extended hiking options back around the lake or down the river.

NEARBY ACTIVITIES

If you want to, you can connect to the Hidden Falls hike. Hidden Falls is a small waterfall cut high into the bluffs of the Mississippi River, above the dam and not all that far north of where the creek from Minnehaha Falls empties into the river. The falls are not visible from above or below, but a short trail leads there from either direction. The flowage is infrequent and sparse, but the little forested cove in which it's nestled offers some solitude along the busy river boulevard. Hidden Falls is accessible from the river trail leading out of Crosby Farm. To reach it from Crosby Farm, continue along the paved trail outside the park entrance and past the marina. There is a gate through which you can walk to connect with a paved corridor to Hidden Falls—a 1.5-mile one-way hike. Taking this optional out-and-back will give you another 3 miles of hiking trail.

#15
Crow-Hassen
Regional Park

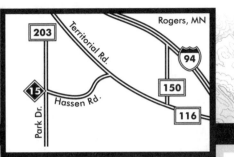

IN BRIEF

One of the biggest prairie restoration projects in the park system, Crow-Hassan features expansive prairies above the slow-moving Crow River. Trails crisscross the meadows and then follow the river for much of its course adjacent to the park.

DIRECTIONS

From the Twin Cities, take Interstate 94 north to Rogers, exit into town, take Main Street (County Road 150) south 2 miles to CR 166, north 2 miles to Hassan Parkway, west 2 miles to Park Road/Sylvan Lake Road (CR 203) north to park entrance on left. Drive to first parking lot on right at the horse trailer staging area.

DESCRIPTION

Crow-Hassan Park offers a full range of natural amenities, from expansive rolling prairie-like grasslands above the river valley to pockets of oaks and other hardwoods scattered along trails that serpentine out-and-back along the Crow River and ultimately return to the parking lot. When I hiked this park, the park map was apparently not up-to-date, since trails designated as hiking-only were also being used as horse trails. Whether this is new policy or not, I'm unsure, but each trail intersection is well marked with a hiker- or horse-icon labeling the appropriate use.

KEY AT-A-GLANCE INFORMATION

Length: 4.6 miles

Configuration: An irregular loop

Difficulty: Easy, mostly flat or gently rolling, with a few steep but short inclines

Scenery: Large expanses of prairie bordered by trees and dotted with lakes

Exposure: Some shade in southern part of the park and along the river; full sun on the prairie

Traffic: Peaceful along prairie trails and river; horse trails can be noisy

Trail Surface: Wide, earthen trail, some mowed lanes of grass

Hiking Time: 1½–2 hours

Season: All season; some designated "ski only" trails in late fall, winter

Access: $5 daily vehicle permit, $27 Patrons Annual Hennepin Parks permit

Maps: Available at park headquarters or at www.hennepinparks.org

Facilities: Primitive with pit toilets and walk-in camping; no water

Special Comments: A good park for a casual stroll—don't be in a hurry; a stop along the river is a must

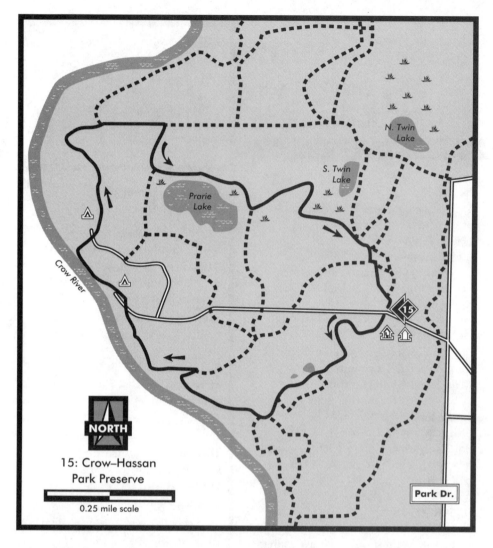

15: Crow–Hassan
Park Preserve

0.25 mile scale

Hiking the designated horse trails presents a challenge: the trails are soft and ground into a fine, almost silt-like texture from all the hooves. This can make walking as tedious as tromping through loose sand. Still, there's opportunity to select several routes as you leave the prairie uplands and make your way along the tranquil Crow River, which forms the western boundary of the park.

Leaving the parking lot just inside the main entrance (also the horse trailer staging area), follow the trail marked "hikers-only" that leads south to the river. Keep on this main trail as it continues to drop to the edge of the river. Along the way, several trails appear on the left; ignore them. Once by the river, the trail turns into a horse trail and follows the river along its northwest/northern bank for about 0.4 mile. About 0.2 mile from where the trail first meets the river, a visible side path down a cut in the embankment leads to the river's edge and a gravel bar (at low water, at least) that stretches for several yards downstream.

This is a great place to stop and view the river, have a picnic, and watch for canoeists paddling by. The Crow River is considered one of the foremost features of the park. Horse and hiking/pet trails follow most of its 7-mile western boundary. Farther downstream is a designated canoe take-out area for access to the park from the river.

Like most parks, Crow-Hassen serves as both a seasonal home and resting spot for scores of bird species on their migration to and from the northern regions. In the fall, the trees along the river are alive with blackbirds—hundreds and hundreds of them. Swans stop over in one of the lakes in the interior of the park.

After paralleling the riverbank for about half a mile, the trail turns sharply for a short but steep uphill climb (about a 20 foot rise in elevation) for the first glimpse of the expansive prairie for which Crow-Hassen Park is renowned. This central prairie and a section further north are part of a 480-acre prairie restoration management area.

The trail levels off as it skirts the prairie and continues along the trees lining the top of the riverbank. A major hiking trail intersects here, and if you've bitten off more than you can chew, you can take this trail through the prairie and back to the parking area.

But most folks will elect to continue along the river, which is bordered by a thick, continuous band of oaks. The surface of this trail turns to pea gravel (the trail is used by horses, too) as it continues along the upper slopes above the river. Ahead is a group camp in the guise of an old farm setting. The trail circles around this bit of development and continues once again along the river. Here the trail passes through another corridor of oaks.

You can enjoy the lushness of summer along these trails through dense corridors of maples and oaks. In comparison, late fall and winter hikers can enjoy an open understory and canopy, once leaves are shed, for long looks through the trees. Some trails look completely different from season to season.

As you circle around to the far western perimeter of the park, some of the trails are more like service roads—wide, grassy, rutted. There are two options for cutting back to the east. One is to stay to the left and follow the outside trail as it loops back at the northwest corner. Another option is to take the road-like lane to the right. This is one of the old Red River oxcart routes used prior to railroads in the area. This is the only section of the oxcart trail that ties into this particular hike, so I decided to take it for a quarter mile to the east, where you can connect with the hiking trail again.

This trail leads trekkers right through the heart of an upland prairie with a mantle of flowing grasses and the occasional renegade tree. An Adirondack-like shelter sits above Prairie Lake. The shelter has a table and a stove for four-season use. The trail follows the north shore of Prairie Lake. The area immediately to the north and northeast is the most complete example of the prairie plant community. In 1968, naturalists discovered an ungrazed and untilled borrow pit, which showed a profile of the undisturbed prairie prior to agricultural use by the early settlers. This led to Hennepin Park's prairie restoration and management efforts in the park.

In the fall, keep your eyes open for large, white birds on the far shore of the lake. You may very well see a few trumpeter swans resting on their journey south along the Mississippi flyway corridor. Other birds to watch for are meadowlarks, grasshopper sparrows, vesper sparrows, pileated woodpeckers (they leave a rectangular hole in dead trees) and red-tailed hawks, probably the most common hawk in Minnesota.

The trail continues along the northern end of the lake and up to an intersection with a service road. Take a right on the service road and hike for about 200 yards to where the hiking trail intersects on the left. Take that left to remain on the hiking loop. For the next 0.7 mile the trail meanders over and through even more prairie as it skirts past islands of aspen, maple, and birch. At about 0.3 mile along this section, South Twin Lake can be seen to the north.

The trail climbs and winds its way back through a small island of trees before gradually climbing up through a wooded area behind the parking lot and horse staging area.

Nearby Activities

Lake Rebecca Regional Park, where paddle and hiking opportunities abound, is only 8.3 miles upstream from Crow-Hassan Park.

#16
Eastman Nature Trail

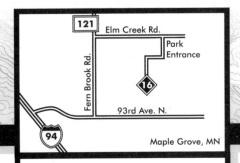

121 — Elm Creek Rd.

Fern Brook Rd.

Park Entrance

16

93rd Ave. N.

94

Maple Grove, MN

IN BRIEF

Eastman Nature Trail lies at the heart of the Elm Creek Park Reserve, the largest park in the metro area. Each lobe of the trail system showcases the best this park offers.

DIRECTIONS

From Minneapolis, head north on Interstate 494. Continue west for about 3 miles, where it becomes I-94 again, to the exit ramp for 93rd Avenue North. Take 93rd Avenue North to the right (east) for about a mile to Fernbrook Lane (County Road 121). Turn left and go another mile to Elm Creek Road. Turn right into the park and follow the road to the park entrance on the right. Continue down toward the Nature Center and park.

DESCRIPTION

The Eastman Nature Center hike is the shorter of two hikes in this book (See Elm Creek, page 60) located in the area's largest metro park. This interpretive trail is a good primer to the diversity of the area's ecosystem, and definitely complements the other, longer hike, should you want to combine the two for a day's worth of hiking.

Begin your hike right out the back door of the Nature Center. Follow the signs to the Meadowlark Trail along a well-marked, wood-chip trail. You will be walking through a dense stand of

KEY AT-A-GLANCE INFORMATION

Length: 3.8 miles

Configuration: Irregular figure eight

Difficulty: A few elevation changes, but basically level and easy

Scenery: Meadows, hardwood forests, ponds, and creek beds

Exposure: Sun and shade intermixed throughout; mostly shade in creek area

Traffic: This is a very popular center but a multitude of paths provide trails for everyone

Trail Surface: Mowed grass, earthen trail

Hiking Time: 1½–2 hours

Season: Probably best enjoyed early spring through late fall. Could turn into a winter wonderland with snow

Access: $5 daily vehicle permit, $27 annual regional park permit

Maps: Available at park headquarters

Facilities: Rest rooms and drinking water at the center

Special Comments: If you're going to take the Elm Creek Trail or others in the more remote reaches of the park, bring snacks and water

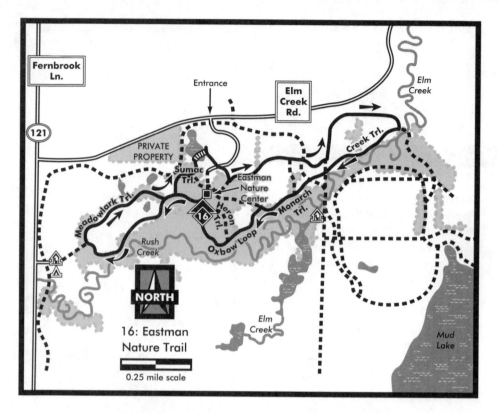

16: Eastman Nature Trail

0.25 mile scale

sugar maples, up a gradual incline to the Sumac-Meadowlark Trail junction. Take the left-hand trail toward Meadowlark.

A short distance beyond this junction, on your right, is a grass pathway that is the Landscape for Wildlife trail. This short interpretive trail explains the practice of planting bushes and shrubs that attract birds and other wildlife. Some of the varieties along this trail and throughout the park include wild plum, hazelnut, and black chokecherry. You will take this trail later when you can use it to join up with the next connecting loop.

Another short distance beyond the Landscape spur, the trail forks again. Stay to the left and walk clockwise around this large meadow along Rush Creek.

The meadow is dotted with young aspen trees. It's also your first introduction to a species that seems to be very prevalent in this park—the prickly ash!

This is a nasty small tree-like plant similar to a young ash sapling in size and appearance. However, the stems and branches have rose-like thorns that can pierce your skin, rip your clothing, and make a most miserable time of cutting through the understory. Prickly ash is common here and in other parks in this part of Minnesota.

The trail has become an earthen pathway through this old meadow that also contains box elder and ash. It winds through a thicket of these species before it comes to a bench that provides a view over the meadow. Soon after the bench, the trail swings down toward Rush Creek and follows it for about a quarter mile. This low-lying area also tends to flood in the spring, judging from the number of sand deposits and grass strands laced throughout the lower branches of the alders growing here.

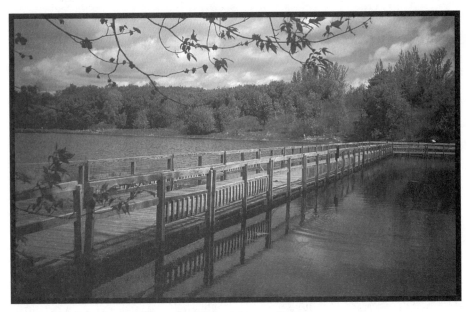

The Boardwalk Trail spans the pond at Eastman Nature Center.

At the top of the Meadowlark Loop, you will come to a trail that leads to the Rush Creek Group Camp. From here the trail swings back into the woods as it rises up perhaps 30 to 40 feet out of the lower meadow-and-creek area along a trail that is again covered in wood chips.

Next, the trail is a grassy corridor through a thicket-like growth of sumac, ash, and box elder. The trail skirts the upland edge of the meadow as it climbs through a transition zone between the lowlands of the creek bed and the upper zone of maples and hardwoods. Basswood trees are more common now as the trail winds through islands of trees and across small meadow-like openings and grasslands.

You will come upon another bench, on the right, that looks down through a narrow corridor of bushes to the meadow below. The trail continues on, cutting through more prickly ash and sumac before opening up on another meadow on the left. If you are hiking in the late spring, about 150 yards beyond the bench on the left, look for the beautiful blooms of a wild crab apple tree right alongside the trail!

The trail passes through an area with marshes on both sides, some with open water. These ponds are great places to watch for migrating waterfowl and summer lake dwellers such as great blue herons and great white egrets.

As the trail swings to the right, you can get a better view of the pond on your right. A few hundred yards later, you return to the previously-hiked feeder trail. Look for the intersection with the Landscaping for Wildlife loop shortly thereafter on your left. Take it.

The Landscape Trail is only a few hundred yards long. It cuts sharply to the right and connects at a T intersection with the Sumac Trail. Take the Sumac Trail to the left and follow the signs to the Boardwalk. You will come upon another intersection with a bike trail marked "to Landscape Trail," but stay on the Sumac Trail and keep heading toward the Boardwalk. Looking through the trees you can see the lake and board-walk ahead, so keep it in your sights.

As you approach the lake, check out this forest. You'll see basswood, maple, and oak. This stand is younger and thick-er than other stands you've been through. It's also the site of branch-breaking, tree-tearing, 125 mph winds that ripped through here in the early 1980s. As you look at the forest floor, you can still see some of the larger trunks of trees that were knocked over during that blast of wind.

The Boardwalk Trail spans the open pond. Step onto the boardwalk quietly and you might see a painted turtle sun-ning itself on the logs and floating mats of debris on the left. It's also common to see summer visitors of Canada geese in ponds and lakes, so check out the far end of this pond while out on the boardwalk.

Upon leaving the boardwalk take the trail to the right, then cross the main park entrance road. Just after crossing the paved roadway, there is a trail to the Out-door Classroom on your left. This is the trail you want to take to continue along the outer interpretive loop of trails.

You will walk right past the classroom circle in a clearing just off the main road. Look for a grassy trail going up a hill at the other end of the open circle. This spur intersects the Monarch Trail to the east. If is the spur isn't readily visible, just stay on the current trail; it, too, con-nects with the Monarch Trail, just a few yards further down. In either case, once you intersect with the Monarch Trail, turn left.

As you wind up and around on the trail you will pass under silver maples and box elders before coming out onto the open meadow. Cresting a knoll, you may see signs of a recent controlled burn

of these grasslands. The burn must have occurred in early spring, 2001. As of the middle of May that year, you could still see the blackened stems and exposed roots of the charred vegetation. The area on the left side of the walkway had been burned earlier, so you can compare the two sides to see how fast it takes for Mother Nature to regenerate after a prairie fire.

The path winds across these meadows as it flows up and down over gentle swells in the grassland. More burned areas appear on the left beyond a bench perched near the highest point on this vast prairie-like area.

As you come down the far side of the meadow, the wide grassy trail forms a right angle intersection (to your right) with a trail that heads back down to the creek. Keep going straight. A few yards farther and you will cross the paved bike trail. If you wish to add the 11.3-mile loop hike through the rest of Elm Creek Park Reserve, turn left here and follow descriptions for Elm Creek (page 60). Otherwise, cross the paved trail and stay on the main course for another 0.1 mile or so until you come to the T intersec-tion with the Creek Trail. Take a left and follow the trail up through the meadow for about a half mile before dropping south to another T intersection. Take the trail to the right along Rush Creek.

You are now heading back to the visi-tor center. The Creek Trail rejoins the Monarch Trail (keep left). You'll be walk-ing under some of the biggest, tallest maples in the park along this corridor. About 0.2 mile farther you will come to another fork in the trail. Keep left again to enjoy the outer loop. This is the Heron Trail. Another 0.2 mile and it will fork again, this time joining the Oxbow Loop. Take the left again and enjoy the bottomlands of Rush Creek. You pass under huge cottonwoods and basswoods in this area.

At a sharp bend in the creek you'll find a bench and short fence defining an observation area. Beyond this point are several wooden footbridges over the creek. This area can be buggy after spring floods. After several bridges, you'll see a series of big birdhouse-like structures. These are wood duck nesting boxes.

The trail rises a bit and the forest becomes maples and oaks again. The trail rejoins the Heron Trail for a short segment before it rejoins the main trail about 50 yards from the trailhead behind the visitor center.

NEARBY ACTIVITIES

The entire park is over 5,300 acres, so the trail network is quite extensive. Options include many more miles of trails both north and south of the Nature Center complex of trails.

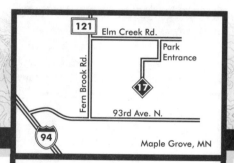

Maple Grove, MN

#17
Elm Creek Park
Reserve

IN BRIEF

King of the trails in this book for shear mileage covered, the Elm Creek Trail offers a grand route through mostly unspoiled Minnesota countryside. There are marshes, hardwood forests, lots of meadows, and plenty of room to stretch your hiking legs. If you've got the time and want to make it a good half day of hiking, this is the trail for you.

DIRECTIONS

From Minneapolis, head north on Interstate 494. Continue west when it becomes I-94 again for about 3 miles to the exit ramp for 93rd Avenue North. Take 93rd Avenue North to the right (east) for about a mile to Fernbrook Lane (County Road 121). Turn left and go another mile to Elm Creek Road. Turn right into the park and follow the road to the park entrance on the right. Continue down towards the Nature Center and park.

DESCRIPTION

With more than 5,300 acres within the park's boundary, Elm Creek naturally offers one of the longest hiking loops in the state. The 10-mile Hayden-Lemans Lake loop encircles most of the northern half of the park. This same area is ground moraine of the Des Moines lobe of the Wisconsin ice age. The combined watershed of this area drains more than 70,000 acres, nearly one-third of Hennepin County. It is through this expan-

KEY AT-A-GLANCE INFORMATION

Length: 11.25 miles

Configuration: A fat, crescent-shaped loop with several side spur options

Difficulty: Mostly flat and even with a few long but moderate grades to conquer

Scenery: A showcase of central Minnesota, from marshes to maples, fields to forests

Exposure: Both shade and full sun, be prepared on hot days

Traffic: Not too crowded once away from the Nature Center complex

Trail Surface: Paved throughout since it doubles as a bike route

Hiking Time: 3½–4½ hours

Season: All seasons; some segments double as ski trails in winter

Access: $5 daily vehicle permit, $27 annual regional park permit

Maps: Available at park headquarters

Facilities: Rest rooms and drinking water at the center; nothing along the hike; you are on your own

Special Comments: Bring snacks and water, few places are designated for rest stops so pick your own along the way

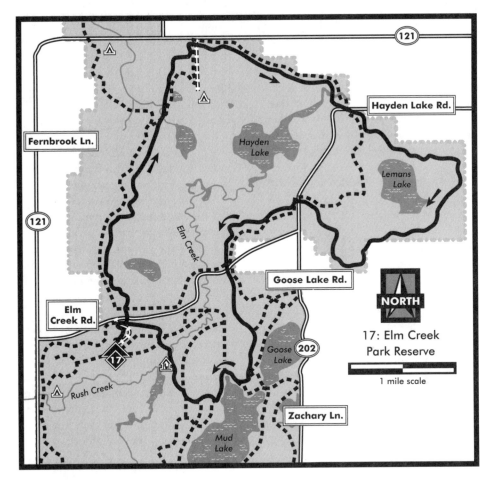

17: Elm Creek
Park Reserve

1 mile scale

sive drainage area that this paved hiking
trail leads.

For parking convenience, start at the
lot at the Eastman Nature Center and
follow the road up to Elm Creek Road
and the park's entrance. From there, go
right a couple of hundred yards to the
trailhead of Elm Creek Trail.

The trail is paved, ten-feet wide and
well maintained throughout the hike. It
starts out along a shallow hog's back ridge
bordered by grasslands. The trail meanders
through the wooded, hilly area. A stand of
maples, with a sumac understory will be
on your right before you cut through a
marsh area with many willows, dogwoods,
and, of course, marsh grasses and cattails.

These are but a few of the many wetland
basins in this part of the park. You'll see
representative cattail marshes, sedge meadows, and tamarack swamps, all bordered by
woodlands or grassy meadows typical of
the more open prairie.

At about 1.5 miles, you'll cross a
wooden foot bridge as the trail continues through marshy areas. There are
some big woods nearby. In fact, a sanctuary of "Big Woods" forest is preserved in
the northwest section of the park—and
not accessible to visitors. Many wild
turkey sightings are reported in this area.
There are also several trail spurs off the
main trail. These are mostly snowshoe
trails used during the winter.

After the footbridge, the horse trail that has been running parallel to the left of the hiking trail crosses over and runs parallel up the right side as the features of the park turn into more open areas with more wetlands. The trail is on a gradual incline at this point. For the next quarter mile it will serpentine its way through alders and dogwoods on the right, and more wooded areas on the left. You are basically skirting the wetlands around Hayden Lake to the east and an unnamed lake nearer you, also to the east.

At the extreme northern end of the main park, the trail runs smack into CR 121 and parallels this road for nearly a quarter mile. There are several parking areas on CR 121 for those who wish to hike only these northern segments.

At the Hayden Lake Group Camp road, hikers are about a third of the way along this loop. The trail follows a power line for this section. It's open country with scattered stands of aspen, some eastern cedars, and open expanses of grasslands.

You will be reminded at the trailhead that there are no facilities along the entire 10-mile stretch. No toilets, no drinking water, and only one picnic table that I saw. There are several places to stop along the way for a light picnic, however. At high noon in summer this trail could become very hot. It's a 10-foot-wide black bituminous surface with shade available only in islands of trees off the trail.

After paralleling the highway, the trail turns abruptly south and crosses a foot bridge at Hayden Creek. If you want, venture up the creek toward Hayden Lake to possibly see a flower for which the area is well known—Minnesota's state flower, the showy lady slipper.

You have several options to shorten your hike at this point. You can take the Lake Road to the right and cut nearly 2 miles off this hike or take the horse trail to cut about 1.5 miles. Both of these options pass through an area listed as having Indian burial mounds. Whether these mounds are particularly discernible or not is something you'll have to discover on your own.

Staying on the main trail past this juncture, you'll cross under the power line again. The trail takes a steep uphill climb just past the power lines at Hayden Lake and then continues along the upland prairie area of the park. Here the path skirts the extreme eastern boundary of the park and the residential and commercial area of the town of Champlain comes into view. Several trail spurs lead into Champlain, where you can access several convenience stores to get some refreshments. There is also a lone picnic table sitting on a knoll at one of these spurs.

Back on the trail, continue on past an unnamed lake on the left (Lemans is on the right), through larger trees in a more mature wooded area with more open spaces. There are more houses along this area, too, but at least now there are mature oaks and maples through which you can walk and not focus on someone's backyard.

The trail climbs out of the lowlands, past more houses and more trail spurs. The trail keeps climbing, slowly but steadily as you go first south, then west. Shortly after the trail turns to the north, you will intersect Goose Lake Road and the horse trail. At this point you are about two-thirds of the way along this trail. Cross the road and follow the trail as it heads west, then slowly curves left to go south. You will intersect Elm Creek Road 0.7 mile after leaving the last road crossing. If you are starting to tire and want to shorten the hike, turn right along the horse trail or follow Elm

Creek Road about 2 miles to the park's entrance. Otherwise, continue south across the road for the last 3-mile section of trail.

Turn right at the next intersection and follow the signs back toward the Nature Center. This takes you along the western shore of Goose Lake. At the southern end of the lake there is yet another intersection. The trail to the left runs between Goose and Mud Lakes and meanders the southern half of the park—that trail is another day's hike in its own right. Instead, head right, following the signs that direct you to Mud Lake. It's about 2.5 miles to the Nature Center.

The trail actually follows a hogback ridge above the northern end of Mud Lake before climbing up along yet another ridge that is lined with sumac, making a nice corridor through which to hike. At the top of the ridge is another lone picnic table with a nice view of the lake. When first approaching, Mud Lake appears to be a marshy wetland only. Rising up to the ridge, you realize that the southern half of the lake actually contains water.

The trail continues along the lake until it intersects with a trail that directs hikers back towards the Nature Center—now only 1.2 miles away. Once on these trails, you will find many spurs that all eventually lead back to the center. Many of these are interpretive trails that the Eastman Nature Trail hike (page 55) explores.

The main trail and the horse trail converge at the creek crossing. This is Elm Creek again, cutting its way across the park. From here, it's a steady uphill climb to the upper meadows just east of the park's entrance. You will come out almost across the road from the trailhead you took 10 miles earlier. From here, it's a gentle downhill loop to the main parking lot.

Nearby Activities

The Eastman Nature Center has such an extensive interpretive trail system that I've chosen it to be a hike onto itself. If you're up to it, there are several more miles of great trails to hike. There's also a route around Mud Lake.

#18
Fish Lake
Regional Park

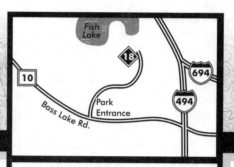

IN BRIEF

Fish Lake and the glacially-deposited ridge offer hikers a setting of shorelines and inclines as this trail winds through oaks and alongside marshes on a short but scenic hike. This is one of those trails that would make a peaceful evening stroll.

DIRECTIONS

Take Interstate 494 north from Minneapolis to US Highway 10 (Bass Lake Road). Go left (west) on Bass Lake Road about a mile to the park entrance on the right. Take the park road into the first parking lot on the left.

DESCRIPTION

This hike encompasses a short network of looped trails that enables hikers to experience this entire park, situated on the southern shores of Fish Lake.

Take the paved bike/hike trail at the north end of the parking lot for the first half of this 2-mile journey. (Ignore the dirt tail starting in the middle of the parking lot.) The paved hiking trail passes a second lot and approaches the visitor center. The bike/hike trail is one-way counterclockwise, so stay to the right of the visitor center. Follow that trail (called the Bay Point Trail) around the knob of the land that sticks out into Fish Lake.

As the trail circles the shore of the peninsula, you'll notice you're at the

KEY AT-A-GLANCE INFORMATION

Length: 2.4 miles

Configuration: An elongated figure eight

Difficulty: Fairly level, easy walking along paved trails

Scenery: Open view of lake, typical Minnesota hardwood forested area

Exposure: Mostly full sun, some shade

Traffic: Multi-use park, most activity around lake development

Trail Surface: Paved

Hiking Time: 1 hour

Season: Park is closed from Nov. 1 through Mar. 30 except for ice fishing

Access: $5 daily vehicle permit, $27 annual regional park permit

Maps: Available at www.hennepin parks.org

Facilities: Recreation area with swimming beach, visitor center, rest rooms, drinking water

Special Comments: Quaint neighborhood park on a lake

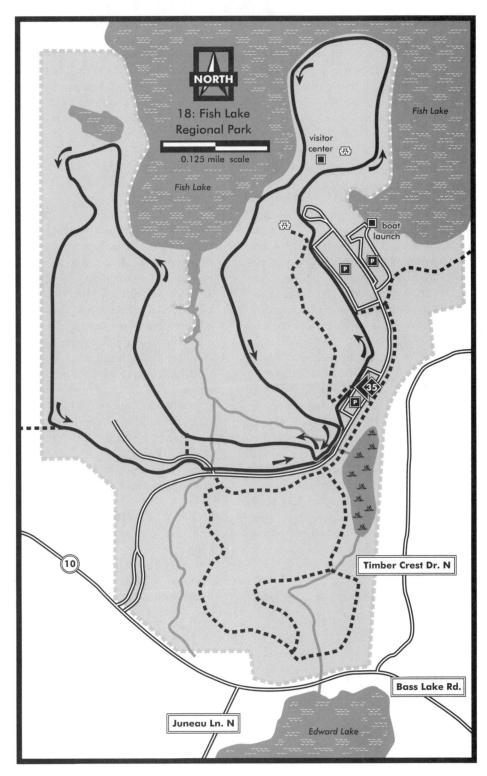

bottom edge of a tree-covered knoll that juts out into the lake. Sumac line the trail, while ash and maples dominate the slopes. Marsh grasses and cattails extend about 30 yards from the trail to water's edge.

As the path turns west, you'll come upon a wooden fishing pier jutting out into the lake. This is also a good viewpoint to look to the north to see the extent of Fish Lake. If not for the park's amenities on shore and the houses across the lake, this could be any of hundreds of quaint lake settings up north. As you continue, the knoll rises to about 40 to 50 feet, atop which grow stately oak trees.

The trail continues its wrap around this knoll, then comes out at the other side of the visitor center and onto the beach area. Continue across the beach to reach the trailhead for the second major bike/hike loop in the park, the Glacial Ridge Trail. (*Note:* Earlier map sources say that the Glacial Ridge Trail is a turf hiking trail. This section, according to signage at the lake, is also called the Glacial Ridge Trail but it is part of the paved bike path.)

After following the shore of Fish Lake for 0.1 mile, the land once again rises some 40 to 50 feet above the lake, though the trail stays level, with a shallow ravine or draw skirting the base of this ridge as the trail continues south. Look across the ravine beyond the marshy area and you'll see another glacial ridge helping to create the valley you are now hiking up. Here you'll see matured oaks and ash lining the slopes of the ridge, while the red twigs of the red-osier dogwood spread out all along the marsh side of the trail.

Just before the main park road comes back into view, a wooden footbridge carries the trail over a small creek. The trail rises slightly and meets up with the main bike/hike trail.

If you're out of time, take a left and return to the parking lot where this trail narrative started. However, if you'd like more wooded areas and more glacial ridges, turn right and continue on the pet/hike loop for an additional mile of hiking. As soon as you cross the creek, take the trail to the right. This trail makes a big loop by first following the other side of the marsh area and creek you hiked earlier, then following the southwest edge of Fish Lake. There is a rest area here for a relaxing break in the hike.

Follow the trail back around and you will come to the main intersection on the main bike/hike trail. There is a spur off to the right as you meet up with the main road. This leads to more trails south of the park entrance road. Stay on the main trail and you will arrive at the parking lot where the trail started.

NEARBY ACTIVITIES

Fish Lake is at the center of a circle of parks that stretch across the northern urban area. Elm Creek is a few miles to the north, Clifton French is a few miles to the south.

#19
Fort SnellingState Park (Snelling Lake and Pine Island Trails)

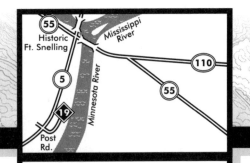

IN BRIEF

Two trails for the price of one! Located between Minneapolis and St. Paul, this hike around Fort Snelling State Park offers a glimpse into Minnesota's history at the confluence of two of her most important rivers—the Minnesota and the mighty Mississippi.

DIRECTIONS

From Minneapolis, take Interstate 494 east to Minnesota Highway 5. From St. Paul take I-494 west to MN 5. Go north on MN 5 to the Post Road exit, the park entrance is on the right. Head toward the visitor center parking area, where this hike begins.

DESCRIPTION

The first part of this hike explores Pike Island and follows a hiker-only trail system that runs along the perimeter of the island. Whether you go clockwise or counterclockwise around the loop, you will intersect two cross trails that offer the option of shortening the hike.

It's a short jaunt from the visitor center parking area to the trailhead on Pike Island. A 0.2-mile spur from the lot cuts through a sampling of the type of growth you will experience throughout this hike. This is river bottomland, a jumble of understory comprised mostly of silver maple, some ash, and a few stately cottonwoods, veterans of many floods.

KEY AT-A-GLANCE INFORMATION

Length: 6.2; 3.3 miles for Pike Island; 2.9 miles for Snelling Lake

Configuration: Two loops, each off a spur from the visitor center

Difficulty: Easy; trail surface varies along level, river bottom terrain

Scenery: Mature stands of river bottom species with continuous vistas of the river or lake

Exposure: Prairie Island shaded; Snelling Lake shaded to the west

Traffic: Popular park; bikes are allowed at Snelling Lake

Trail Surface: Pike Island is earthen and mulch; Snelling Lake is mostly paved with some gravel

Hiking Time: Pike Island, 1½–2 hours; Snelling Lake, 1½ hours

Season: All seasons; cross-country skiing/snowshoeing on Pike Island

Access: Minnesota State park fees—$4 daily, $20 annual permit, $12 annual pass for disabled persons

Maps: Available at park or www.dnr.state.mn.us/parks_and_rec reation/state_parks/fort_snelling

Facilities: camping, visitor center, drinking water, rest rooms

Special Comments: Occasionally the park closes due to high water; call (612) 725-2724 for information

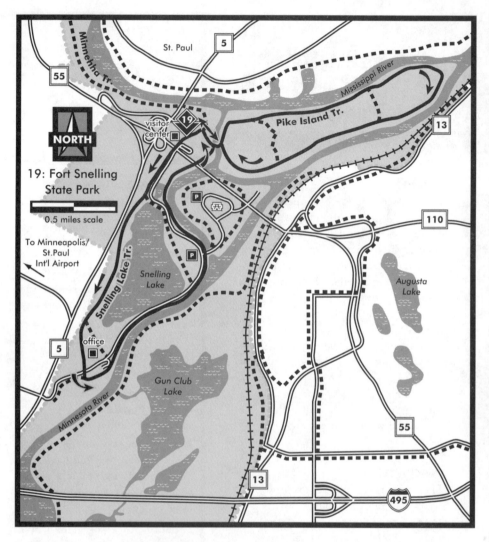

The path leads to the bridge connecting the island to the main shore. You can follow the Hiking Club Route to the right or take the other path to the left. Either way, both trails lead to the tip of the island at the confluence of the Minnesota and Mississippi rivers—the most geologically significant feature of this historic park. Deposits left during the last Ice Age were subsequently cut with great drainages by massive water runoffs as these newly-created valleys emptied out. Millennia of scouring by these rivers has created the high bluffs and expansive flood plains you see today.

The path follows the river along its banks and through a great understory of towering, broad-based cottonwoods. Some of these incredible trees are at least five feet in diameter at their bases. The fissures in the rough bark measure over four inches deep! About halfway down the southern edge of the island, you may notice sizable gouges in the trees. These are from large slabs of river ice slashing at the bark during periods of especially high water following thaws.

Zebulon Pike, for whom the island is named, came upon this island in 1805 as part of a scouting party to establish forts along the upper Mississippi. Prior to Pike's exploration, the area was first settled by the Dakotas who once lived throughout Minnesota. The Dakotas believed the two rivers were the origin of life and joined to form the center of the earth.

Pike Island is typical of many islands formed by numerous braided channels throughout the course of the Mississippi River, particularly in the northern states. Cottonwoods, silver maple, elm, ash, and willow are the dominant trees throughout this entire region. Floodplains in more-frequently flooded areas will have much less understory than those where flood waters only occasionally reach. Expect bugs and mud in the spring and early summer.

After you complete the loop, head back across the bridge to begin the more civilized hike in the park. The trail around Snelling Lake doubles as a bike trail and is for the most part a smooth, paved surface. It's a great way to see the rest of the park and to enjoy yet another stretch of the river.

From the visitor center, follow the Von Bergen Trail south for 0.3 mile to where it connects with the bike/hike trail at the north end of Snelling Lake. Following the lake shoreline around the western edge of the triangular-shaped body of water, the trail skirts along the bottom of the bluff line that defines the boundary of the park. The trail continues on around the south tip of the lake. There are two trails that lead off to the left from this main trail (either one takes you back to the main park road). Take the second trail to the left through a marshy area and a bridge over a creek draining out of the lake and continue back to the main park road. Go across the park road and continue on for another 0.2 mile and you will meet up with the river trail. This will take you along yet another stretch of the Mississippi for three-quarters of a mile along a paved bike/hike path.

Just as you reach the eastern tip of the lake the trail leaves the lake. There is a fork in the trail—you can continue straight ahead along the gravel trail and follow the river back to the visitor center (with a side trip to a small island connected by a bridge on the right), or you can cut to the left, remain on the paved trail, and go back across the park road to continue along the lake again, past the beach and fishing pier. Once you pass the fishing pier, its a short backtrack to the visitor center.

The park has a sampling of wildlife, from white-tail deer to a harmless but imposing fox snake that resembles the rattlesnake. Birders will enjoy the Snelling Lake Trail, especially the southern end where it's marshy. Along the river, look for great blue herons, egrets, and other shoreline birds.

NEARBY ACTIVITIES

First and foremost is a trip to historic Fort Snelling. Summer programs feature period costumes by staff and in-depth historical information on the area. The trail systems that connect with Fort Snelling include the Black Dog Trail from the south along the river and the Minnehaha Trail from the north and west. Nearby Crosby Farm Park (see Crosby Farm Park, page 47) adds yet another historic perspective to this heritage-rich area of Minnesota.

#20
Frontenac State Park
(Bluffside Trail)

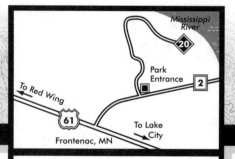

IN BRIEF

One of my favorite parks, Frontenac offers exceptional trails along some of the steepest bluffs in the area. (Though this route can be made into an out-and-back, if the bluff line hike is too difficult.) With more geological and cultural history than parks three times its size, Frontenac State Park is truly a hidden treasure, well worth the drive south of the Cities.

DIRECTIONS

From the Twin Cities take US Highway 61 south. Frontenac is 10 miles south of Red Wing. Turn left (east) on County Road 2 and go about a mile. Entrance is on left. Drive to end of road and park.

DESCRIPTION

This is one of those parks with such a fantastic history that you are compelled to learn about it before you take to the trails. Knowing an area's geological beginnings and the cast of players who helped make the region's history adds to the personality of any site, and this one in particular.

Hundreds of millions of years ago, Minnesota was covered by a shallow sea. Sediment accumulated at its bottom and slowly changed into rock. That rock is now visible as the bluffs of the Mississippi River. In glacial times a gigantic river, called the River Warren, was fed from glacial run-off. It carved the giant valleys through which many of Minnesota's

KEY AT-A-GLANCE INFORMATION

Length: 2.5 miles

Configuration: Short loop coupled with an elongated loop

Difficulty: Difficult along 400-foot bluffs with steep ravines and intersecting trails; switchbacks help

Scenery: Impressive valleys, overlooks, mature stands of oak and maple, open meadow atop bluffs

Exposure: Fully exposed meadows atop bluff, dense canopies in ravines

Traffic: A park known well by locals, but a mystery to many

Trail Surface: Grassy lanes to narrow trails cut into the slopes; slippery in spots when wet

Hiking Time: 1½–2½ hours

Season: All seasons, but steep trails best in summer

Access: Minnesota State Park fee system—$4 daily, $20 annual permit, $12 handicap/annual.

Maps: Available at park or at www.dnr.state.mn.us/parks_and_recreation/state_parks/frontenac

Facilities: State park amenities—campsites, rest rooms, showers, etc.

Special Comments: I've driven past this park for over twenty years. —my mistake!—great hiking and incredible scenery and history

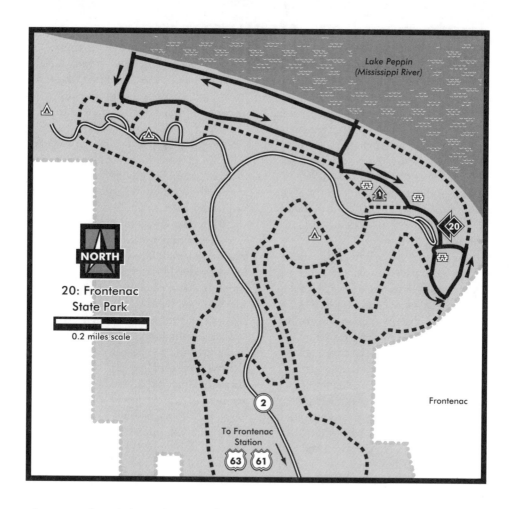

NORTH

20: Frontenac
State Park

0.2 miles scale

20

Frontenac

To Frontenac
Station

63 61

2

rivers now flow. At its peak, most of Frontenac was underwater—except for the park's bluff.

In more recent historical times, archeological digs at Frontenac in 1976 uncovered artifacts from the Hopewellian culture dating from 400 B.C. to A.D. 300 Some of these sites were burial grounds; others indicated that the tribes lived in the area as well.

Dakota and Fox Native Americans later settled in this valley, followed by French explorers who might have actually built the first church in Minnesota here. The famous French missionary, Father Louis Hennepin, led the first

European exploration to this area of the Mississippi River in 1680.

In 1727 an expedition left Montreal to set up a post in this area in order to launch further exploration westward in search of a route to the Pacific Ocean. The French-Indian War caused these settlements to be abandoned until the mid-1800s, when the first permanent pioneers settled.

By the 1870s, Frontenac was enjoying status as a premiere tourist destination—a resort town—drawing visitors on riverboats from as far downriver as New Orleans. Looking out over this valley today, with views of trains along the river, small towns and farmsteads, and forested bluffs, you can truly sense the spirit of this area.

A number of trailheads leave from various points along the parking lot. This hike starts out with the short, but intense, Interpretive Trail loop off the eastern end of the main picnic area parking lot. Having a map handy at the onset is advisable because of the trail options available. Whether you tackle the full extent of the Bluffside Trail or the much less strenuous meadow network of trails, you owe it to yourself to take this loop first.

The interpretive trail packs the essence of the entire park into a short, dense, looped trail. Trailheads are not always marked, but the maps available are accurate. The start of the trail is well-marked and beckons hikers with a groomed, three-foot-wide grassy lane through aspens and oaks. Several trails extend off this pathway to the right, including one about a 0.1-mile spur from the parking lot trailhead. Marked as the Observation Point Trail, it leads to a beautiful overlook of the valleys to the south and the old town site of Frontenac.

Back on the main interpretive trail, the path descends over the top of the bluff line and literally down into the geological history of the park. The bluff now behind you used to be the only point of land in an inland sea that covered all of what is now the great Mississippi Valley. With their steep, 400-foot embankment still below you, the sandstone bluffs provides a narrow line for this path to follow.

Along the way, mature paper birch, sugar maple, and huge cottonwoods guard the banks. There is a moderate understory below you and a wall of worn sandstone standing like a fortress on your left—some of this exposed rock reaches thirty feet high.

This area is known as Garrard's Bluff, named after the founder of Frontenac, General Israel Garrard. Riverboat pilots named the same area Point No Point because of the optical illusion that it was a true point of land when viewed from upriver.

Evidence of quarry activity can be found in a few of the iron rings still solidly fastened into the ground near the quarry site. This rock was of high quality and favored by many architects. The Cathedral of St. John the Divine, in New York City, is made of Frontenac limestone from this quarry. Imagine the restraints needed to lower massive blocks of limestone down the steep 400-foot embankment to waiting barges on the river below!

At about this point the trail intersects with a steep trail dropping to the right and away from the base of the bluffs to the river banks below. Take this trail, and then go left at the river. Continue for another 1.1 miles before heading back up to the top of the bluff. The Mississippi River at this point broadens into the start of Lake Pepin. By the time the river reaches Lake City, about 5 miles to the south, it's over 3 miles wide.

This area along the river is renowned for bird-watching. Both the river area and the upper bluffs are visited by passing species during spring migration. Frontenac's bottomlands are famous for a variety of warblers. The hardwoods in the bottomlands create a perfect nesting habitat for the prothonotary warbler. Be watchful along the river during spring and fall migration for sanderlings and ruddy turnstones, two shorebirds that travel between South America and the Arctic each year! Bring your bird book and binoculars, as over 200 species have been sighted here and throughout the park.

The segment climbing back up towards the top of the bluff is 0.3 mile and leads up to a T intersection at the base of the bluff. At the T, there is a short spur to the left. This leads to a distinctive natural landmark—a huge rock with a hole in it positioned close to the edge of the bluff. Called In-Yan-Teopa in the language of the local Native Americans, this massive rock outcropping may have had some religious significance.

A short trail spur leading back from the rock puts you back on the bluff trail. Return to the intersection and continue left, which brings you to the observation platform above In-Yan-Teopa. Take a left to continue along the base of the rocky bluff. Otherwise, the trail straight back from the observation deck leads up to the edge of the campground where a second trail follows along the top of the bluff—also leading back to the main parking lot.

However, stay on the lower of the two trails. As you advance along the base of the rocky ledge, you will see two short spurs to the right that head up to the campgrounds. Stay on the main trail for the next half a mile, then you will come to an intersection with a third trail. This trail crosses the bluff trail from its trailhead at the picnic area atop the bluff on its way down to the river. If you take the right fork at this intersection, you just parallel the trail you are on, as they both continue for 0.2 mile back to the steep switchback staircase at the end of the interpretive loop that will take you up to

the top of the bluff and back to the parking lot at the picnic area.

At the top of the switchbacks is another observation deck with fantastic views of the Mississippi River Valley. The trail rejoins the picnic area and the parking lot at the opposite end of the interpretive loop near where you started.

This hike only scratches the surface of the trails available here. Additional hiking opportunities exist south of the picnic area. Those trails wind across and along upland meadows all along the bluff tops, after which they again drop down into the ravines on the back side of the river bluffs. The northwest loops of the trails cut through the walk-in camping area and create a network of trails along the grassy meadows between the ravines. A 1.5-mile loop drops down one ravine, follows the park road, and then climbs back up another ravine to the bluff-top meadows along the upper road system and the developed area of the park.

NEARBY ACTIVITIES
I'd have a hard time leaving this park, but a trip to old town Frontenac is worth a visit. If you are a golfer, one of the prettiest and most hilly courses in the area is right across the road at Frontenac Golf Course (for tee-times call (651) 388-5826 or (800) 488-5826). They have incredible vistas on top of bluffs even higher than those at Frontenac State Park.

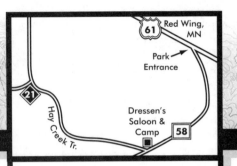

#21
Hay Creek
(West Trail)

IN BRIEF

Hay Creek offers one of the more demanding hiking opportunities of all the parks near Minneapolis and St. Paul. Comparable to some of the steeper terrain found in the bluff country along the Mississippi River, Hay Creek's deep-cut ravines, white pine plantations, and mountain foothill–like switchbacks provide a moderate challenge for hikers.

DIRECTIONS

Drive south from Minneapolis/St. Paul to Red Wing. Take County Highway 58 South about 4 miles to Hay Creek (turn right at Dressen's Saloon & Campground onto Hay Creek Trail). Go 1.4 miles to the first parking area past the picnic area on the right and immediately over the bridge on the left. West Trail is at the end of the dirt parking area.

DESCRIPTION

The Hay Creek unit of the Richard J. Dorer Memorial Hardwood State Forest is an equestrian's park. Attempts to keep some of the trails reserved for just hiking have not worked. Horses are ridden along every trail in the park to the point that the DNR has decided to bow to this pressure. Older maps still show "hiking only" trails, but they are a thing of the past.

Hay Creek is not technically a "park" but rather a "management unit." It was one of the first blocks of forested land to

KEY AT-A-GLANCE INFORMATION

Length: 1.6 miles

Configuration: A multi-lobed balloon

Difficulty: Moderate, but with a nearly 250-foot rise in elevation; some parts level and easy

Scenery: Deep ravines and mature hardwoods; some plantation pines give it a northern boreal forest feel

Exposure: Mostly exposed, but full shade in plantation

Traffic: Trails shared with equestrians, but these are the least used

Trail Surface: Packed earth throughout; nice, wide pathways

Hiking Time: 1–1⅓ hours

Season: All seasons—the only trail section closed to snow mobiles; good snowshoeing in winter

Access: No fees to hike

Maps: State Forest Map and fold-out Management Unit maps available through DNR; no on-site information

Facilities: None, this is a minimally developed management area

Special Comments: A short hike with nice views across the valley to give an illusion of high elevation hiking; take left trail at fork for easiest uphill climb

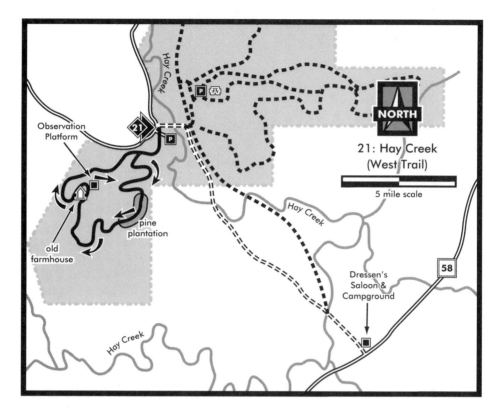

Observation
Platform

21

P

NORTH

21: Hay Creek
(West Trail)

5 mile scale

Hay Creek

pine
plantation

old
farmhouse

Hay Creek

Dressen's
Saloon &
Campground

58

Hay Creek

be purchased in Goodhue County after the state established the Richard J. Dorer Memorial Hardwood Forest in 1961. This forest is a patchwork of wooded areas that stretch from just south of Hastings to the Iowa border, following the Mississippi River and stretching westward nearly 50 miles in pockets of hardwoods throughout southeastern Minnesota.

The land was eroded, poor-quality farmland in need of conservation recovery. Its trout streams and scenic bluff country made it valuable recreational land. By 1970, over 1,500 acres had been acquired in the Hay Creek Management Unit alone.

The primary forest trees include a variety of oaks, with elm, birch, basswood, and black cherry mixed in. In areas along the many creeks and a few of the larger washes, cottonwoods, willow,

and soft maple dominate. There are also a few plantations of walnut and pine scattered throughout the unit.

Almost every type of conservation management practice has been used at Hay Creek. There have been timber sales, tree plantings, and various timber stand improvement projects. Old fields are now pine plantations. You can see their green canopies across the valley from various points along Hay Creek's West Trail.

There are actually three major hiking areas within the unit. The northernmost unit contains multiple-use trails are available for hiking, skiing, horseback riding, and hunting. These hills have trails that cut alongside ravines, encircle the edges of fields, and follow washes back down. Of the 25+ miles of trails looping around Hay Creek, over 20 miles are in this section alone. This is probably the most concentrated use area in the park and the most heavily used by equestrians and therefore not a high priority on my list during heavy summer use.

A second unit leads off the picnic area and follows a ravine for a 2.5-mile loop. This trail, once designated as a hiking-only trail, has been receiving more horseback use lately according to DNR officials and other hikers.

This hike explores the third area, a trail less traveled by equestrians and the only trail loop on the opposite side of the road from all the other activities. It's a short 1.6-mile loop, but offers the diversity of forest types, deeply-cut ravines, and gains in elevation that are comparable to those areas of heaviest use. It also features two fieldstone structures worth visiting.

The trail begins beyond a gate and a vandalized, metal trail map (full of bullet holes!). The trail is a simple balloon loop out-and-back so a map is not really needed for directions. The first section is an unassuming corridor through the trees.

Follow this corridor for about 0.1 mile to a small stand of spruce trees. The trail then turns to the left and after a short distance comes to a fork, the start of the loop. If you go right its about a 0.5-mile hike up a steady rise in elevation of over 270 feet. However, if you take the left fork, you gain the same elevation through a series of casual switchbacks and intermittent sections of level terrain. Either way you end up back at this fork. The hike description below follows the left fork.

The first section of this trails climbs about 60 feet into a maple-and-aspen corridor. The angle of the trail, the degree of slope, and the somewhat open trees all blend together to give one the sense of hiking up a trail in the foothills of the mountains. If you look over your shoulder along this section, you'll see across the valley floor the curved, ravine-etched slopes of Hay Creek Valley and the plantation-capped hilltops and goat prairies common to this area.

Birch and aspen saplings grow beneath scattered, taller oaks. At about 900 feet in elevation, the trail switches back in the opposite direction and continues climbing. It continues through more gnarly oaks.

The trail switches back, for the third time, as you approach the top of the ridge. Ahead of you is one of the many plantation plantings done after the purchase of the area. With a smattering of white birch among the white pine, this area has a northern boreal forest look to it. The trail meanders through this dense stand of pine trees for about a quarter of a mile. The trail appears to be following the top of the ridge, but the map shows the course slightly lower. In any case, it's a beautiful corridor through a stand of pines I would estimate being about 60 to 70 years old.

Exiting this pine stand, you skirt an upland meadow and reach the halfway point on the trail. The elevation here is about 1,060 feet (the parking lot was about 840 feet). The trail maintains this elevation for about another 0.2 mile while it meanders along the edge of the meadow and the upper edges of the steeply cut ravines that begin at the lower end of the meadow and drain into Hay Creek.

After skirting the open meadow, the trail cuts back into the woods. Check out the tall trees with the black, scaly bark. These are wild cherry trees.

A word of warning: This trail, too, has been relinquished to horseback riding. It's very narrow in this section, so consider stepping off the side of the trail when riders pass.

The trail climbs back up a bit and turns to the right. At this bend are the remains of an old stone work shed. Its made of flat stones and mortar. Just beyond it at the top of the incline is an observation platform. Be very careful climbing the steps, it appears that the beams supporting them could give way anytime. The view, even from ground level, is of the entire Hay Creek to the east. The open patches near the tops of the hills are called "goat prairies," because the area's of open grass are so steep only goats could graze them. The dark green caps on the hills are plantation plantings of pines similar to the one you just hiked through earlier in this segment.

As the trail continues back to the ridgeline it immediately passes a stone farmhouse. Built of squared off stone, the walls of the house rise two full stories to a peaked roof. A foundation with cellar make this stone edifice over three stories high. Some of the early construction techniques are still readily visible.

The trail now begins a gradual but steady descent to the intersection at the fork in the trail near the parking lot. From about 1,050 feet down to 860 feet, the trail meanders gracefully through the forested area. The wooded area thins out, the aspen and birch are more sapling sized, and the airiness of the trail allows you to look out over the valley again.

You rejoin the trail stem beyond the fork and return to the parking lot.

NEARBY ACTIVITIES

Great trout fishing in Hay Creek, more trails in the northern section. Nearby Red Wing offers shops, the riverfront and another great hiking experience along Barn Bluff.

#22
Hyland Lakes Park Reserve (Richardson Interpretive Trail)

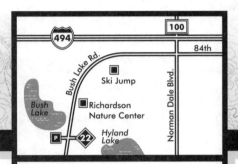

IN BRIEF

Hilly islands of oak and aspen inter-mixed with some representative prairie meadows and dotted with ponds throughout a rather short network of hikes in the less-developed portion of the park.

DIRECTIONS

From Interstate 494 and Minnesota Highway 100, go south on MN 100, which becomes Normandale Boulevard. Continuing south to West 84th Avenue, turn right and cross County Road 28 to where 84th becomes East Bush Lake Road. Follow road south, past the entrance to Richardson Nature Center (on the left) and continue another 0.4 mile to the Bush Lake parking lot on the right. Access to the southern loop of the network is across the road, to the left of the trailhead for the Pet Trail.

DESCRIPTION

Though the park has over 11 miles of trails open to hikers, I selected this hike because it is in the least-developed part of the Hyland Lakes complex. The Bush Lake parking lot provides access to a number of trailheads. The paved pet/bike trails begin their 5-mile loops here and takes pets, pedestrians, and pedalers in a circle around the open prairie and nes-tled hills in the center of the park.

However, to get a better sense of the wild side of this country, this hike follows

KEY AT-A-GLANCE INFORMATION

Length: 2.1 miles

Configuration: A series of loops, accessed by an out–and–back from the visitor center or a short spur from Bush Lake parking lot

Difficulty: Easy to moderate; hilly, and meandering in wooded areas

Scenery: Winding paths through stately oaks, glimpses of ponds through the dense understory

Exposure: Fully shaded woods to open-sky prairies—evenly divided

Traffic: These trails are fed only by visitor center guests

Trail Surface: Wide, mulch-covered pathways through woods and mowed lanes through meadows

Hiking Time: 1–1½ hours

Season: All season: access to some trails may be restricted in winter

Access: $5 daily vehicle permit, $27 Patrons Annual Hennepin Parks permit

Maps: Available at visitor center or at www.hennepinparks.org

Facilities: Visitor center offers rest rooms and drinking water

Special Comments: This is a very expansive park with fully developed facilities, yet most nature-oriented trails are confined to a small area

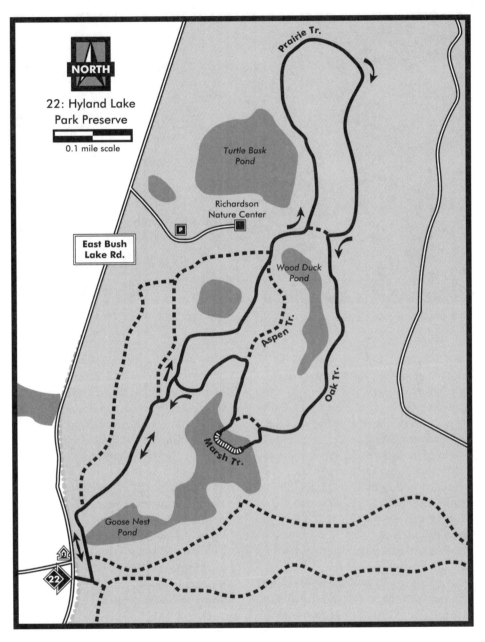

22: Hyland Lake Park Preserve

NORTH

0.1 mile scale

Turtle Bask Pond

Richardson Nature Center

East Bush Lake Rd.

Wood Duck Pond

Aspen Tr.

Oak Tr.

Prairie Tr.

Marsh Tr.

Goose Nest Pond

some of the trails that loop out from the Richardson Nature Center and provide one with more samples of oak and aspen woodlands and restored prairie than do other areas of the park.

Park in the Bush Lake parking lot and go to the trailhead right across the high-

way. This is the start of the pet/hike trail. However, immediately to the left is an unnamed trail spur that heads left (north) from its intersection with the paved trail. About 200 yards up this wide, mowed pathway through the prairie grass, you'll come to a fork in the

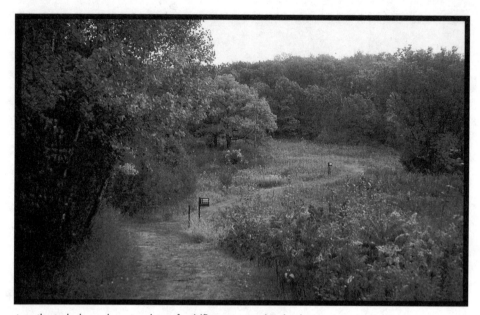

A trail winds through a meadow of wildflowers at Hyland Lake.

road. Take the trail to the right. This pathway undulates through the hilly meadows surrounding Goose Nest Pond visible on the right. Expect to see Canada geese from the trail leading into the wooded area ahead.

This pond is one of a half dozen scattered throughout the park—mostly concentrated in this area—totaling more than 80 acres. Coupled with over 150 acres of wetlands (mostly to the west around Anderson Lake) these water habitats attract a wide variety of birds and other wildlife.

The trail climbs gradually to an island of aspens growing on the hills adjacent to this meadow. This is part of the Grantsburg and Superior lobes of the Wisconsin glaciation that occurred over one hundred centuries ago. The hills are evidence of deposits that were later sculpted and scoured into lakes and hills and valleys. Over 30% of the entire Hyland/Anderson/Bush Lakes area has a soil make-up that causes it to retain and hold

water instead of allowing it to drain away.

From the Aspen Trail, cut back into the forested area at the sign for the Oak Trail and enjoy a canopied walk through mature burr, white, and red oaks typical of the upland oak woodland transition zones so common to this part of Minnesota.

I hiked this trail in the fall, just as leaves of understory vegetation were starting to fall. In denser stands of trees, this opens up vistas not readily seen during the summer. It also makes bird-watching easier as winged critters flit from branch to branch just ahead of intruding hikers. Nuthatches, chickadees, and flickers were ever-present in this section.

The trail continues in a winding northerly direction past several smaller ponds. These are populated in the fall with several varieties of ducks, many of which are preparing for the long-haul migrations south. One small pond had quite a number of the beautiful, multicolored wood ducks, the ever present mallard, and several Canada geese that pass through the Twin Cities every season.

From the classic oak woodlands, the trail continues northerly to the open prairies between the Richardson Nature Trail and the steep slopes of Mt. Gilboa, a 1,020-foot "mountain" rising out of the woodlands. This is where the Hyland Ski Area development is located. Hyland has about 46 acres of restored native prairie. Some of the prairie has been reclaimed from the agricultural fields that were created long before this area was park land.

Expect a profusion of wildflowers during late spring and early summer on the trail loop that cuts through this meadow for about 0.7 mile. There are also some small islands of sumac in this area, particularly along the southern portions of the meadow loop, that are striking in full fall coloration.

If you go counterclockwise around this loop you will come back around past Turtle Basking Pond. Its a typical marsh-fringed pond replete with tall, dead tree snags, rushes, and duck weed. Chances are good that you will see one of the indigenous turtles basking on a log jutting out on the pond's surface. The park lists prairie skinks, Cooper's Hawks, pileated woodpeckers, bluebirds, and tiger salamanders as some of the main fauna observed in the park. Walking silently along the many ponds is certainly a good way to see many of these and other critters.

If you were to start your hiking at the Nature Center, you would be entering the loops at a point just south of this pond. An alternative route back to the starting point would be to take the long loop south into the southern meadows near the trailheads accessible from the Bush Lake parking area.

More can be enjoyed by continuing back down the outermost eastern loops. You will come back into the oak woodlands, back along more rolling hills and wide, shaded corridors. You'll pass yet another pond, a long and narrow pond called Wood Duck. If you continue on along the west side of Wood Duck Pond, you will come back to the open meadow. You are now at the southeast end of the loop and even closer to Goose Nest Pond. A wooden observation platform allows you to step right to the edge of the pond and observe the activity going on.

The trail then follows the upper edge of the basin, along the meadow and back down the eastern side to the trailhead across from the Bush Lake parking lot.

NEARBY ACTIVITIES

Bring your mountain bike. More than 5.6 miles of bike trails have been developed in the southern half of Hyland Park.

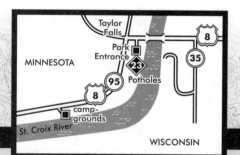

#23
Interstate Park, Minnesota

IN BRIEF

Walk along expansive river bluffs, a for-mer railroad grade, and along one of the world's largest glacial potholes in the Minnesota section of this century-old interstate park. Vistas of the St. Croix Val-ley and environs round out the sites that help complement the activities found across the river.

DIRECTIONS

From Minneapolis, take Interstate 35 West north, from St. Paul, take I-35 East or US Highway 61 to Forest Lake. At Forest Lake take US 8 toward Taylor's Falls. At the intersection with Minnesota Highway 95, turn left (north) to Taylor's Falls. At the intersection just as you are turning right to cross over bridge into Wisconsin, take a sharp right into the potholes area of Minnesota's Interstate Park parking lot.

DESCRIPTION

Though Interstate State Park is now protected, at one time this and the sur-rounding areas provided a valuable resource for the logging industry. With vast tracks of white pine to the north and a wide river to float them down, the logging industry soon proved to be an economic boon to Minnesota and neighboring Wisconsin. As Taylor's Land-ing grew and the area became increas-ingly popular with visitors, many people started building in the Dalles section of the St. Croix. Recognizing that the

KEY AT-A-GLANCE INFORMATION

Length: 0.3 mile along potholes section trails; 3.8 miles along river and railroad bed for total of 4.1 miles

Configuration: Loop with spurs

Difficulty: Mostly easy or moder-ate, with rugged sections along river

Scenery: Great geologic features and fantastic views of the river

Exposure: Mostly sun, some shade

Traffic: Potholes always attract vis-itors and even rock–climbing classes; trails used more by campers

Trail Surface: Some constructed walkways at potholes, earthen trails with exposed roots and rocks

Hiking Time: 2–3 hours, includ-ing time wandering potholes

Season: Mostly summer, haz-ardous in most areas in winter

Access: Potholes open 8 a.m. to 10 p.m. daily; $4 daily vehicle permit, $20 annual regional park permit

Maps: Available at park or at www.dnr.state.mn.us/parks_and_ recreation/state_parks/interstate

Facilities: Rest rooms, visitor cen-ter/gift shop, drinking water at pot-holes, boat launch, campground

Special Comments: Minnesota side offers more potholes in small area and a longer hike on the river

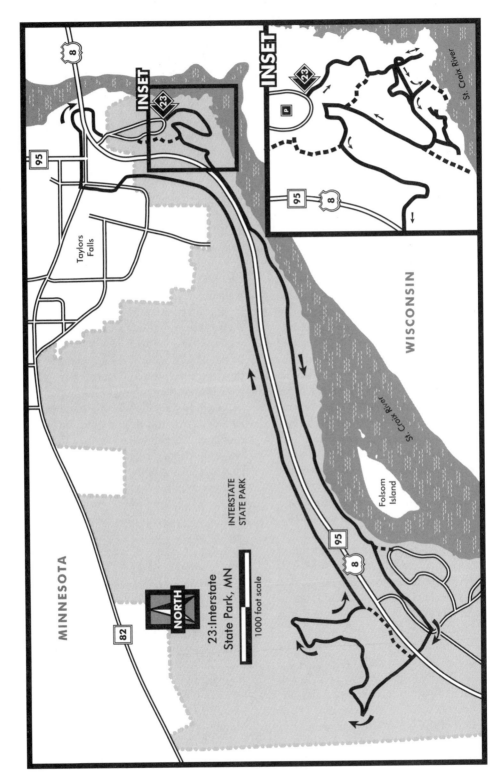

INSET

INSET

St. Croix River

23

P

23

95

8

WISCONSIN

St. Croix River

8

95

Folsom Island

INTERSTATE STATE PARK

23:Interstate State Park, MN

1000 foot scale

NORTH

MINNESOTA

82

Taylors Falls

95

8

beauty and unspoiled nature of the land was threatened with continual development, a bill was introduced and passed in 1894, authorizing the state to work with Wisconsin to acquire land along the river. Over 1600 acres were set aside between the two states, and Interstate State Park became the first interstate park in the United States.

Before you start, go to the visitor center right at the entrance to the parking lot to see the small museum. When you are ready, find the paved pathway beyond the state park office and visitor center at the opposite end of the parking lot from the museum and begin.

The first part of this hike explores the park's amazing potholes, one of which, the "Bottomless Pit," is said to be the deepest explored glacial pothole in the world. The route from the visitor center begins just beyond the building and leads down a paved pathway over basalt layers laid down over 11,000 million years ago. You can see the force of erosion from flowing water with sand and boulders churning in it. Smooth and wavy formations and myriad potholes ground into the hard rock all attest to the power and the persistence of time.

Forget following any prescribed hike (though certainly follow the route I've plotted on the map if you want guidance), and instead, wander around this area until you are satisfied you've seen everything from every angle. This is more like a pre-hike, but will be worth it for the opportunity to walk amid these huge boulders and outcroppings and to get occasional glimpses down to the river and across to Wisconsin from the edge of the bluff. The pothole network is only about 0.3 mile long, but meandering could add another 0.1 mile to this segment.

Part of the trail is self-guided and takes visitors past the Bottomless Pit, the Bake Oven, and the Cauldron. There is even a

tight L-shaped crack in the rock called the Squeeze. It'll confirm whether or not that diet of yours is actually working.

There are also two spur trails that lead to observation platforms above the river. During the summer, you should see canoers and kayakers plying the waters below. One of the observation decks is immediately across the river from a popular rock-climbing face on the Wisconsin side of the Dalles. The first of these two observation platforms also allows you to look upstream and down. This right-angle bend in the river is a result of glaciated waters flowing into and then being diverted by a fault line in the basalt. The water, taking the path of least resistance, turns sharply to the right to form this acute bend in the river.

After spending time at the potholes, you take on a 2.75-mile loop that leads to the Minnesota state campground downstream. To reach this trail, head back toward the parking lot using the main, paved trail and take the trail to the left across the road from the drinking fountain. The trail leads you up a short but steep climb to the highway before cutting back to the left to parallel the roadway atop the slope above the river.

The trail passes through the highway overlook and continues to the campground and picnic area about 1 mile downstream. The trail climbs and dips along the banks of the St. Croix. Be sure to wear good scrambling shoes along this primitive trail.

At about 0.75 mile from the trailhead, just before you approach the campgrounds, you will come to a fork in the trail. The left fork takes you through the campgrounds, but you want the right fork, which continues past the campground to the information office at the campground entrance.

To the left of the office is a trail spur that heads up to and under the highway via a concrete, six-foot-tall tunnel. Immediately afterwards, you'll come to a T intersection. Continue to the left and follow the signs to the ancient waterfall along the 1-mile Sandstone Bluffs Trail. This trail heads past the massive footings from the old train tracks and up the valley to an "extinct" waterfall. It then climbs the bluff, passes two observation points, and drops back down to join up with the Railroad Trail. If you don't want the extra 1-mile climb, turn right at the T and follow the Railroad Trail back to town.

The railroad came to Taylor's Falls around 1880, long after it had developed as a popular tourist retreat and well into the establishment of the lumber industry that took millions of board feet of white pine out of the area.

This is a straight shot, as railroad right-of-ways tend to be. It's a tree-lined corridor through maples, oaks, and upland hardwood understory. The trail ends at a parking lot behind the Taylor's Falls Community Center, a modest white-sided building a few blocks from the pothole park section. Continue out to the street. A small schoolhouse, Minnesota's oldest standing schoolhouse, will be on your left as you head to the right down to the next street intersection.

Take a right again and cross Bench Street, this is the main street feeding into downtown from the highway on the right. Cross the street and head to the left of the entrance onto the bridge. The pathway takes you under the bridge to the right and back up to the entrance to the parking lot at the potholes.

NEARBY ACTIVITIES

Wisconsin's side awaits, and the town of Taylor's Falls is a cool tourist town. Riverboat tours are given throughout the day during the summer and many outfitters in the area rent canoes and gear for paddling on the St. Croix.

#24
Interstate Park, Wisconsin

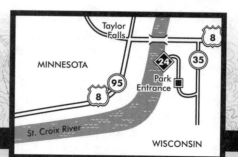

IN BRIEF

Hike through sections of the United State's oldest interstate park, exploring the many billion-year-old geological formations scattered along the trail. This hike complements the interstate hike in Minnesota, offering excellent views of the St. Croix River and 23-acre Lake O' the Dalles.

DIRECTIONS

From Minneapolis, take Interstate 35 West north. From St. Paul, take I-35 East or US Highway 61 to Forest Lake. Take US 8 toward Taylor's Falls. Continue across the bridge into Wisconsin and go uphill to Wisconsin Highway 35 and take a right at the sign to Interstate Park. Continue south to the park entrance. Stay on the park road to the second right. Park in the spaces adjacent to the intersection with North Campground Road.

DESCRIPTION

The Interstate Park hike on the Wisconsin side begins at the second right after passing the park entrance. The sign at the intersection says "North Camp Ground." Turn immediately to the left into one of the few spaces in front of the pine trees.

Interstate Park is part of the "National Ice Age Reserve"—nine units stretching from Lake Michigan to the St. Croix valley. It's an area rich in geological evidence of the ice age 10,000 years ago

KEY AT-A-GLANCE INFORMATION

Length: 4.6 miles

Configuration: Irregular figure eight with one out-and-back spur

Difficulty: Easy-to-moderate; some steep grades, uneven footing

Scenery: Breathtaking vistas and shear cliff overlooks

Exposure: Sunny along Dalles, shady in maple forests behind bluffs

Traffic: Very popular day destination; hosts rock-climbers in summer

Trail Surface: Uneven earthen path, exposed boulders, roots, narrow and hilly in some areas

Hiking Time: 2–3 hours

Season: Early spring to late fall; slippery and hazardous in winter

Access: $5 daily for Wisconsin residents, $7 out-of-state; annual pass $18 for Wisconsin residents; $25 out-of-state

Maps: Available from park office at entrance

Facilities: Picnic area and shelter, bath house, rest rooms, showers and swimming area at lake, amphitheater, fishing pier, camping, Ice Age Interpretive Center and Gift Shop

Special Comments: More trails than on Minnesota side; bring your camera

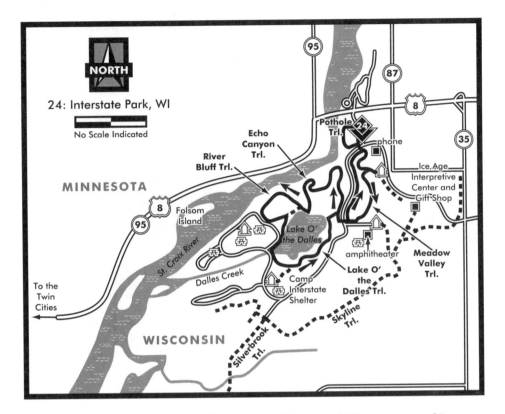

NORTH

24: Interstate Park, WI

No Scale Indicated

MINNESOTA

Echo Canyon Trl.

River Bluff Trl.

Pothole Trl.

phone

Ice Age Interpretive Center and Gift Shop

Folsom Island

St. Croix River

Lake O' the Dalles

amphitheater

Meadow Valley Trl.

To the Twin Cities

Dalles Creek

Camp Interstate Shelter

Lake O' the Dalles Trl.

Skyline Trl.

WISCONSIN

Silverbrook Trl.

that covered most of the upper midwest in mile-thick ice. The one exception is this area of Wisconsin that was spared the last ice advance. The Dalles of the St. Croix are spectacular reminders of this period.

The modest parking area for the Pot-hole Trail is the starting point for a series of looped hikes that ultimately combine to form a winding trail through huge boulder fields, lava flows, and glacier features. Leave your car behind and follow the trail west as it snakes through huge boulders and around scattered pine trees and stunted oaks on its way to the bluffs above the river. The trail inches its way to the edge of the bluff, about 50 feet to the river below, then turns to the right over a wooden footbridge. The foot-bridge leads the hiker over not a chasm in the rocks, but one of the large pot-holes cut into the hard, rocky bluff.

About one billion years ago, this very spot was being covered in lava oozing out of the ground about 100 miles north of the Dalles of the St. Croix. Thousands of cubic miles of lava covered this area. So massive, the weight of the lava sagged in the middle making a gigantic basin—that basin eventually filled with water. Today we call that expanse of water Lake Superior.

Later Pre-Cambrian and Cambrian layers of sand and gravel from ancient seas were deposited over this lava. Between then and about one million years ago countless rivers and streams cut through the sandstone exposing the lava below. Erosion over eons scraped and smoothed the lava, sometimes cutting channels through it.

About one million years ago, the first of many ice ages advanced on the area, which further contributed to the sculpt-

87

ing of the landscape. One result of the ice age are the many circular pits or holes seemingly bored into the lava. These potholes were formed when a boulder or rock got caught in a depression or crack in the lava. Unable to be washed away, the rock continued to tumble around and around in these depressions. Sand and smaller rocks would get washed into the holes as they were continually scoured deeper and deeper by the grinding boulder. Some of the resulting potholes are over 60 feet deep and nearly 10 feet in diameter. Many smaller ones can be found scattered throughout the rocks here and across the river in Minnesota.

Leave the potholes and continue along the top of the bluff admiring spectacular views of the river. Rock climbers enjoy these bluffs and the trail passes a popular rappelling spot on the nearby bluff top. Shortly after the trail swings to the right, there is an observation platform offering a grand view down and across the river.

The trail intersects several spurs—all leading to points along the edge of the bluff. The designated trail climbs up to a knob that overlooks the park road to the right. At this point it swings back down and to the left and back to the pothole trailhead.

Back at the parking lot, cross the park road to reach the trailhead for Horizon Rock Trail. The map shows it as a 0.5-mile linear trail but don't worry, you're only taking it halfway as a short but rewarding side trip. Head into the woods along a creek bed and through an overstory of maple. At about 0.2 mile you will come to a path to the right. Don't take it yet, continue straight up the slope to the top, another 0.1 mile. Here you will come to steps in the rocks and a large rock knob. Follow the trail up around the knob to the left and you will come to a stone shelter. From the top of

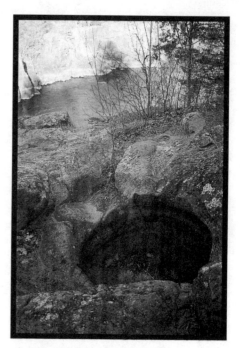

Along the Pothole Trail, the work of volcanoes and glaciers is evident.

the knob is a grand view of the surrounding St. Croix River valley to the south and a bird's eye view of the town of Taylor's Falls to the north. It's a quick and easy side trip.

Descend back to the trail intersection and turn left onto the Meadow Valley Trail. Take this trail for 0.4 mile until you come to a park road at the parking lot for the amphitheater. Take the road to the right out to the main park road and turn right again. Across the road on the left (about 150 yards) is the parking lot for two trailheads: the Summit Rock Trail and a trail to beach house at Lake O' the Dalles. This hike continues along the Summit Rock Trail at the north end of the parking area.

The trail winds through ironwoods as it meanders its way to the bluff line. At about 0.1 mile the trail intersects the Echo Canyon Trail on the left. Continue straight on the Summit Trail through a

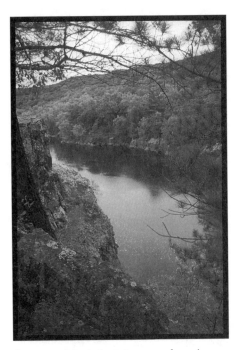
The serene Mississippi river seen from the Interstate Trail.

section that winds through large boulders as it climbs towards an observation deck on the bluff. The deck is a few yards off to the right on a trail spur immediately before climbing up onto the bluff's edge. You can see the river and the tourist river boats that tours up and down the Dalles.

After the observation deck, take the steps up and over the lip and then back down more steps to a second observation deck. The trail follows along and through more boulder fields as it climbs along the bluff line. The trail tops a knoll dotted with short, gnarly oak trees. The trail to the left is not the designated trail—stay to the right and continue on around the knoll.

You will soon come to a trail intersection on the right. This is another junction with the Echo Canyon Trail. Now you can take a right and continue on the Echo Canyon loop. This is yet another loop that winds through boulders and

hardwood forest on the bluff top. About 0.1 mile after the **T** intersection, the trail cuts to the right. It drops down and becomes a bit more rough and rocky. The rock outcroppings in this area reminded me of an ancient, man-made stone wall, complete with seams between the blocks of rock. The trail continues down a steep incline to the cliff edge above the river.

You will pass spurs off this section of the trail that have been closed, presumably to allow for regeneration of the trails. Echo Canyon Trail turns away from the river as you approach a large rock wall. The trail then heads up a valley-like canyon flanked by stately evergreens.

This trail comes out at the shore of Lake O' the Dalles. The **T** intersection offers you a chance to go left towards the bathhouse and the start of this section of the trails at the parking lot. However, to continue hiking, turn right at the **T** and head back for more boulders, maple overstory, and views from the bluff.

About 100 yards down the lakeshore, the River Bluff Trail veers off to the right and up into the woods. You'll pass a small bog on your left and gain a little elevation as you ascend toward more boulder outcropping before approaching the top of the bluff again. There are more open vistas of the river as this trail circles around and drops down a moderately steep, sloping trail that comes out at the River Picnic Shelters Road.

At the bottom of the trail, just as it hits the level park grounds, there is a small deer trail to the left that will take you back to Lake O' the Dalles. Take the left and continue along the deer path, through the understory at the edge of the woods, and you will come out at a **T** intersection at the lake's shoreline. Take a right, follow the lake around to its southern end, meet up with the park road to cross over the creek, and continue along the eastern shore of the lake. This is the Lake O' the Dalles Trail, part of the 1-mile loop around this 23-acre lake.

The first intersection leads back to the Camp Interstate Shelter. Stay to the left for about another 0.4 mile until you come to the beach house. Turn right to follow a section you passed earlier, then stop at the parking lot and intersection with the park road. Either hike 0.5 mile up the park road to get your car, or backtrack along the Meadow Valley Trail again.

NEARBY ACTIVITIES

Besides other great trails in this park, there is Interstate Park's Minnesota twin across the river. Well worth a visit, too.

#25
Kinnickinnic State
Park, Wisconsin

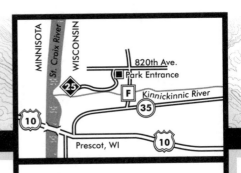

IN BRIEF

One of many rivers flowing into the St. Croix on the Minnesota–Wisconsin border, the Kinnickinnic River offers a hot trout fishing stream, long sandy river banks, and a mix of hardwood forests and restored prairie meadows to hike through on this small piece of Wisconsin countryside.

DIRECTIONS

From South St. Paul, go south on US Highway 10 to Prescott, Wisconsin. Take Wisconsin Highway 35 North (left) up the hill and then turn left (north) on County Road F for about 5 miles to 820th Avenue. Turn left and drive for 0.2 mile to park entrance on left. Follow road all the way to end by picnic area.

DESCRIPTION

The Kinnickinnic River is one of many that flow down from Wisconsin's unglaciated western boundary into Minnesota's border rivers such as the Mississippi, and in this case, the St. Croix River. Renowned as an active trout stream, its fast-flowing waters push sediment out into the St. Croix, where it settles to form the Kinnickinnic delta, reducing the width of that river's channel by half. It was the mouth of this river that first drew attention to this area as a prime candidate for a Wisconsin park.

Soon after the first series of Wisconsin parks were established, the mouth of the

KEY AT-A-GLANCE INFORMATION

Length: 3.2 miles

Configuration: Loop

Difficulty: Mostly level, easy

Scenery: Bluff tops and meadows, surprisingly few glimpses of the river

Exposure: Mostly full sun, some shade

Traffic: Mostly trout fisherman on the river, swimmers on the beach and delta area

Trail Surface: Mowed grass, earthen

Hiking Time: 1–1½ hours

Season: All seasons, would be good cross-country ski trail

Access: $5 daily for Wisconsin residents, $7 out-of-state; annual pass $18 for Wisconsin, $25 out-of-state

Maps: Available at Park Information Kiosk at end of parking lot

Facilities: Drinking water, pit toilet, picnic area, swimming beach

Special Comments: Swimming in the St. Croix is very popular here

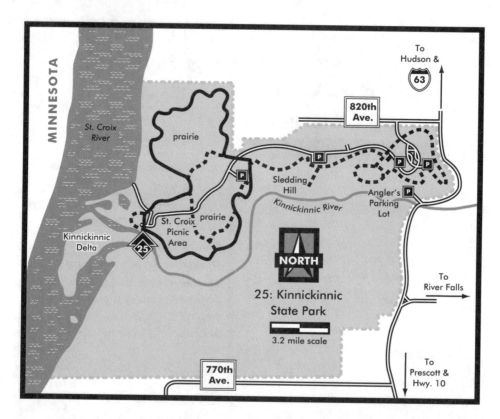

Kinni' River, as the river is called, was among several chosen as future park sites. However, little was done for many decades. As the Twin Cities began to encroach upon the natural areas of eastern Minnesota, concerned landowners began a process to protect the area around the Kinni' River. Parcels of land totaling 45 acres were donated to secure the prospect of a Kinnickinnic State Park. The Wisconsin Department of Natural Resources was impressed by this show of support and the park was established in 1972.

Since then over 20,000 trees have been planted by volunteers and over 50 acres of prairie have been restored. Bird watchers should note that over half of the birds listed for Wisconsin have been found in this park; more during migration. Even in winter this a good place to spot birds; because of the flow of the

water from the Kinni' into the St. Croix, the river around the delta doesn't freeze, making it a natural gathering area for bald eagles in the winter.

This hike is a series of connecting trails forming a loop that showcases those uplands and bluffs that make up this river's character. Each trail is marked with colored, banded posts that correspond to the color guide on the trail map.

The hike begins at the west end of the parking lot, following a paved path past the picnic areas to an impressive overlook above the Kinnickinnic River, right where it spills into the St. Croix below. Retrace your steps to the Purple Trail which leads off to the right as you are coming back from the overlook. Follow the top of the bluff line along the picnic area before heading into the woods. These woods are typical of upper bluff forests in this part of Wisconsin: oaks and maples with some ash mixed in. The understory is dense and lush as the trail meanders through a narrow corridor framed by branches and foliage.

At about 0.4 mile the trail intersects the Orange Trail. Take the right fork and continue along the wooded bluffs high above the river. Below are the swift, clear-running, trout-filled waters of the Kinni' River, popular with fly fisherman who like the wide stretches as it runs through the park. The trout is the "exceptionally large" German brown trout. The Kinni' is a Category V trout stream which means there are certain restrictions and daily bag limits. You must also have a valid Wisconsin fishing license (or out-of-state license) to fish this river.

The Orange Trail wanders for about 0.2 mile before it intersects the Yellow Trail. Stay to the right and continue on the Orange. You are skirting one of the restored prairies of the park at this point. Continue on another 0.4 mile to the intersection with the Blue Trail, which leads east toward a series of trails around the park entrance. Save those for a side trip and instead take the left fork, which is now considered the Yellow Trail. This will cross the park road just to the east (right) of a parking lot at the prairie area.

Over 140 species of birds have been identified in the park and it's estimated that upwards of 90 species could be seen at any one time during spring migration. Also, about 140 species are known to nest in the nearby valleys. This represents about 50% of Wisconsin's nesting bird species. Wild turkeys were reintroduced into the park in 1989—albeit this is approaching the northern limit of their natural range.

This hike continues into the prairie meadows for about another 0.1 mile until you intersect the Green Trail. Turn right to follow this 1.4-mile trail that loops around the northern section of the park, skirting the prairie and more of the upland woods common to the park. It rejoins with the Yellow Trail about 0.1 mile before the Yellow Trail crosses the park road. However, at about 100 yards beyond the intersection with the Yellow Trail (just before the road), there is a trail off to the right, the northern end of the Purple Trail. The Purple Trail parallels the park road and skirts the bluff above the swimming area before joining up with the picnic grounds where this hike started.

NEARBY ACTIVITIES
Trout fishing in the Kinnickinnic River; scenic drive along Wisconsin bank of St. Croix, north to Hudson, south to Prescott.

#26
Lake Byllesby
Regional Park

IN BRIEF

Formed by a dam on the Cannon River, Lake Byllesby is surrounded by open meadows with a few low, moist areas and a small creek that becomes a wetlands just before emptying into the lake. This hike is very low key and relaxing.

DIRECTIONS

From the Twin Cities take MN 52 south to County Road 86 near Cannon Falls. Go west on CR 86 and turn immediately to the left onto Harry Avenue. Take Harry Avenue south for 1.5 miles. Follow this road right into the heart of the park. Parking lot for main complex is on the left. Trailhead is across from the camp store.

DESCRIPTION

Formed as the reservoir behind a dam, Lake Byllesby offers a city park–like atmosphere in the open prairie-and-farm region of southeastern Minnesota. The park has been developed for multiple day-use activities centered around the lake and part of its shoreline.

The hiking trail is a serpentine loop around the undeveloped northern two-thirds of the park. Broad, mowed-grass walkways wind in and out of a random growth of eastern red cedars, most of which are ten to twelve feet tall. These trees block long vistas but are spread out enough to give a sense of openness. In some spots, these trees are more dense,

KEY AT-A-GLANCE INFORMATION

Length: 2.2 miles

Configuration: Loop with many lobes

Difficulty: Very easy, all flat

Scenery: Mostly open meadows with young cedar trees throughout, some plantation planting

Exposure: Sunny throughout, most trees too short to give much shade

Traffic: Casual strollers, most activity around lake

Trail Surface: Mowed-grass pathway

Hiking Time: 1 hour

Season: Mostly three seasons, although it could be hiked or snow-shoed in winter

Access: Fees for camping or shelter rental

Maps: Possibly in park, also at: www.co.dakota.mn.us/parks/byllesby

Special Comments: Expansive development along lake, with modest trails through meadows and wetlands

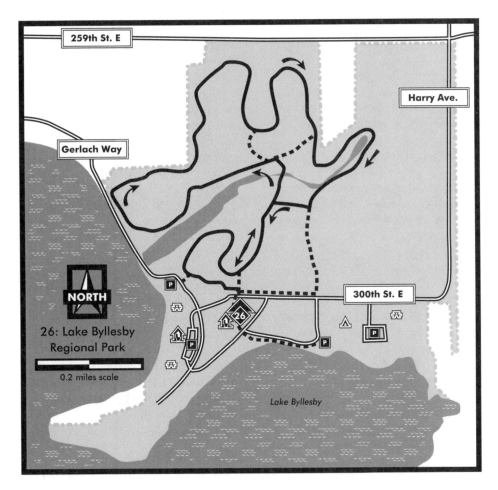

NORTH

259th St. E

Harry Ave.

Gerlach Way

NORTH

26: Lake Byllesby
Regional Park

0.2 miles scale

300th St. E

Lake Byllesby

creating a corridor reminiscent of a big, outdoor maze.

Starting from the main visitor area, walk across the park entrance road to a point immediate opposite the camp store and service area. This is the main trailhead for all the loops to the north. Take this trail into the maze of cedars and roughly 80 yards in you will come to a T with the main loop trail. Take this to the left for a clockwise trek around the entire hiking-trail system.

At about 0.1 mile you'll come to a side spur to the left that accesses the boat launch parking area. This is an alternate starting point if it's too crowded at the main service area. From this intersection

the trail meanders around and almost turns back on itself as it follows the long, narrow marsh area that cuts through the western two-thirds of the park. This loop is about 0.4-mile long and will come back to a spur on the right that connects with the trailhead. Stay to the left and continue on about another 0.2 mile until you come to the footbridge over the open water of the marsh. Just before the bridge, you will intersect a trail to the right. This is where the northern loop of the trail comes back out. Ignore this trail, instead take a left and head toward the bridge.

You may stay drier wading across the water than using the bridge. As of early spring 2001, it was in need of support—if it is still sagging when you visit, test it carefully before crossing.

Once across the creek, the trail comes to a junction. Continuing ahead bisects the two northern loops, but you want to turn to the left. Along the way you'll enjoy some close-up views of the marsh area through the dense growth of alders, willows, and red-osier dogwoods. A dense stand of sumac and what looks like a plantation planting of trees (ash?) marks your halfway point along the marsh. As the path jogs to the left, notice the huge clumps of Amur maple. These can turn brilliant crimson in the fall. Their tiny winged seeds look like the ones you see on maple trees, only smaller.

The trail approaches a road (Gerlach Way) that fringes the lake then turns north. You'll parallel the road for only about 0.1 mile, then turn right. As the trail continues east into the heart of the park there are several group plantings of columnar buckthorn, locust, white pine, and others that seem to have been planted there as landscaping. Beyond the trail to the left is an agricultural field. This trail follows the outline of the park boundary and meanders along the northern block of park land.

At the bottom of the second loop, the trail intersects the trail from the bridge you crossed earlier. Stay on the main trail and continue for another 0.3 mile to enjoy more of the open grass fields and sparsely placed cedars. As the trail heads south it parallels some private residences. At the end of the 0.3-mile section, there is another trail intersection, this one to the right, that returns to the footbridge by following the wetlands area adjacent to the creek. Stay straight and pass the intersection on the right.

From this intersect to the next junction—the last leg of the trail—you'll travel about 0.4 mile. You will come across one last intersection, a trail that heads off to your left. If you don't want to cover ground you've already hiked, you should take this 0.2-mile trail to 300th Street Southeast (the one you came in on), turn right and head back to your car. Otherwise, pass it by and stay in the woods, on this trail, until you come back to the main artery you took at the beginning.

NEARBY ACTIVITIES

Nearby parks offer more trails: Miesville Ravine, Rice Lake, Singing Hills, and Nerstrand Woods are relatively close.

#27
Lake Como, Como Park

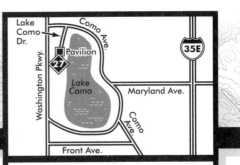

IN BRIEF

Lake Como offers one of only a few hikes right in the City of St. Paul—fortunately it's around one of its most popular lakes. The proximity to other major attractions within the same park boundary makes this hike an easy one to create a plan around.

DIRECTIONS

From Minneapolis take Interstate 94 North to Minnesota Highway 280, exit at Larpenteur Avenue and go east to Lexington Parkway. Turn right (south) to connect with East Lake Drive on east side of Como Lake. Alternative route is to take I-94 East into St. Paul and take the Lexington Avenue exit north to Como Avenue Turn right on Como into Como Park, follow road and signs to Lake Como. From St. Paul take Maryland Avenue west from I-35 exit or Lexington north from I-94. Easy access is also from Larpenteur Avenue to Lexington Avenue intersection. South on Lexington to park.

DESCRIPTION

Como Park's always drawn visitors from beyond its hometown of St. Paul. With amenities such as golf, a zoo, and botanical conservatory, Como provides a pleasant setting via a sprawling, boulevard-laced parkland. In planning a hike around Lake Como, save some energy to enjoy the zoo and the conservatory. By

KEY AT-A-GLANCE INFORMATION

Length: 1.75 miles

Configuration: Loop

Difficulty: Easy, casual walking, no hills, no rough spots

Scenery: Open view of entire lake, surrounded by a variety of landscape trees

Exposure: Mostly full sun, very little shade

Traffic: A popular lake for walking

Trail Surface: Fully paved, 10-foot-wide path around entire lake

Hiking Time: 30–45 minutes

Season: All seasons—sidewalk is maintained throughout winter, too

Access: No charge for parking, free access to pathway

Maps: None on site; try www.stpaul.gov/depts/parks/

Facilities: Rest rooms, drinking water, picnic area, small restaurant on grounds

Special Comments: This is a typical "city park" lake, not a lot of special sights or scenery, but a pleasant place for a casual walk

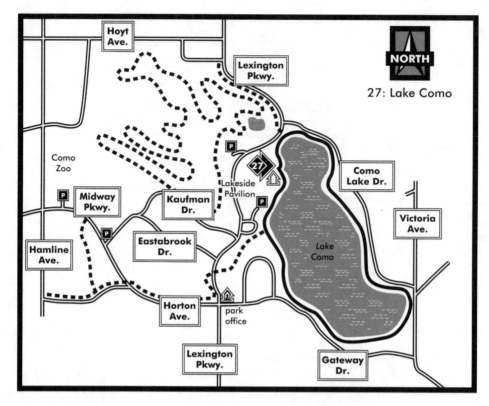

NORTH

27: Lake Como

comparison, the fauna and flora around Lake Como will be very modest. Still, it's in a peaceful, casual setting—just right for a light stroll or brisk walk-workout.

The grand Como Pavilion is the focal attraction on the lake from any angle or point on the trail. It's a big, rectangular bandstand enclosed by tall columns on three sides. It's pretty impressive from any view along the trail around the lake. It's a natural place to begin a hike.

Start from either parking lot as there is one on either side of the pavilion. It really makes no difference which way you go around the lake. Whichever way you choose, make sure you at least visit the man-made Hamm's Memorial Waterfall. It's directly behind the pavilion. It seems slightly out of place, but stretch your imagination a bit and take in the illusion of the north woods and a cascading river.

Facing the waterfall, head left back down to the front of the pavilion and head south (right) along the path that circles the lake. It leads down along the shoreline and up and over a knoll about 0.3 mile from the starting point. Cottonwoods and elms flank the paved, ten-foot path as it continues along the lake.

About one-third of the way around the lake, at about 0.6 mile, there is a dock that extends out about 20 feet from shore. Kids might enjoy fishing for sunfish off its outer edge. Another 0.2 mile and a knoll of pines comes into view on the right. This could be a good spot to sit back and enjoy the view down the long axis of the lake.

A bit farther past this knoll the path leaves Como Avenue and follows Gateway Drive and enters a short corridor of trees. There are a few evergreens in this area. Those with the orange-hued bark are scotch pine. Smaller scotch are popular as Christmas trees. Many of the plantings around the lake are decorative landscape plantings, which will bloom in the early spring, making this a multi-season promenade of tree colors.

The pathway heads north along the shoreline that is lightly trimmed with reeds. Landscape plantings of crab apples and other spring flowering decorative trees continue down the stretch of this boulevard. The lakeshore remains open in spots to offer hikers great views across the lake towards the stately pavilion on the other side.

Almost a mile around the lake the otherwise straight-running shoreline makes a turn to form a rounded point. Its boulder embankment makes the shoreline rather imposing from the water but from shore it's an appealing, open lawn knoll with a few trees and park benches. It is immediately across from the Pavilion at this point. This would be a great spot to sit and listen to concerts or to just see the activity across the way—all lit up at night.

A third parking lot comes into view right after this bench area. These are handy because there is no parking anywhere along the boulevard that parallels the pathway. Residential side streets offer additional parking but one of the five parking lots would be a better choice. These are small but there are enough of

them and you can start the circle around the lake at any point.

The north end of Como Lake borders on Lexington Parkway. The pathway parallels this street for a while before turning back toward the pavilion. This end of the lake has remained open most winters to help concentrations of ducks and geese.

Back at the pavilion you can relax and view the lake from the large second story grand room. In years past you could rent small paddle-wheel craft for a quiet pedal around this end of the lake. There is also a small concession area. The lake pathway is lit by old-fashioned street lamps to make this a perfect after-dinner, light-hiking option.

NEARBY ACTIVITIES
Como Park Zoo has been completely redesigned into a more open environment for viewing the animals (the old drab cages can still be seen in one building). A small midway of rides and full-service concession stands make the area seem like a county fair. The botanical greenhouse conservatory is right next door to the zoo and features exotic plants and colorful blooming flowers year-round. Both places are within walking distance from Lake Como, although not via marked pathways. Better to drive to the zoo and see these features either before or after your hike around the lake.

#28
Lake Elmo Park Reserve, Eagle Point Lake

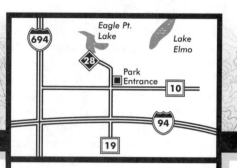

IN BRIEF

Mostly wetlands and forests, Lake Elmo Park features two main lakes, open meadows, and more types and numbers of evergreens than most area parks. This trail keeps the lake in sight for most of its length, while still taking in some of the park's rolling meadows.

DIRECTIONS

From Minneapolis or St. Paul drive east on Interstate 94 to County Road 19. (Exit 251). Go north on CR 19 for 1 mile to park entrance. Follow road into park to first parking lot on left, go to end of parking lot for main trailhead.

DESCRIPTION

Access Eagle Point Lake from the central trailhead in the park's first parking lot.

Leaving the marsh grasses and cattails behind, take Trail 19 uphill into the stand of upland oaks and maples. One of the first things that stood out to me about this park was the number of evergreens—spruce, cedar, white pine—that grow in clusters throughout the entire area. You are heading south, so stay on this trail and continue past the intersection with Trail 17 on your left. You want to stay on Trail 19 through these uplands and around the south end of the lake. You will find more oaks, maples, and ash growing as little wooded islands in the meadows. Most of the meadows are bordered by rows of trees, mostly pines.

KEY AT-A-GLANCE INFORMATION

Length: 3.7 miles

Configuration: Irregular circle following elevation around the lake

Difficulty: Easy throughout, with a couple of minor elevation changes

Scenery: A patchwork of meadows surrounding a marsh grass–lined pond; very picturesque—a sunny, summer day is the best time for this park

Exposure: Mostly full sun, except for wooded area around trailhead

Traffic: Moderately busy in summer and fall

Trail Surface: Medium wide, mowed grassy lanes

Hiking Time: 1½–2 hours

Season: All seasons; very wide ski/skate-ski trail in, winter

Access: $4 daily; $20 annual; reciprocity with Carver and Anoka County parks

Maps: Available at park or at www.co.washington.mn.us/parks

Facilities: Campground with electricity, rest rooms, showers, picnic area, playground, swimming at Lake Elmo

Special Comments: Lake Elmo is a popular boating/fishing lake

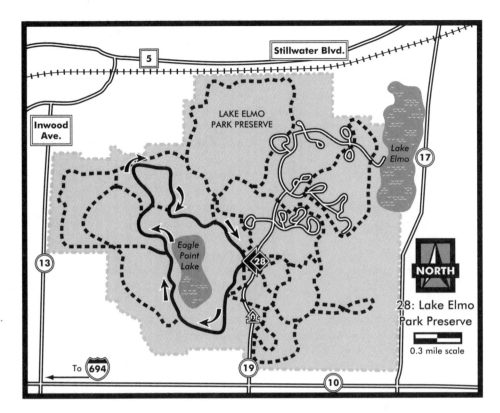

Located close to a major freeway (I-694), this park has a constant buzz from that traffic. Open meadows are particularly susceptible to such ambient noise, as are any of the smaller wooded areas that have lost their sound-buffering leaves late in the season. Fortunately, this is the only section of the hike where that traffic hum was even noticeable. Mature paper birch, maples, and cottonwoods grow throughout this section as do a few fine-needled white pines.

Continue around toward the western edge of the lake, where hardwoods give way to open grasslands characteristic of the oak prairie. It is hilly country sprinkled with wildflowers and edged with spruce. Some of these trails double as horse and cross-country skiing trails. This trail has a gravely surface—soft, but noisy.

Eventually you will come to the Trail 30 junction. It cuts to the left away from the lake. Ignore any signs and take the right fork to continue around the lake. You may still see a lot of downfall from wind damage, as you follow the trail toward the lake. Eagle Point Lake is shallow with many stretches of shoreline thick with marsh grass. The entire lake covers 143 acres and because it is so shallow, it does not support fishing.

The trail continues through an older growth of hardwoods as it gains elevation. Soon it reaches a high point overlooking the lake. A large ski shelter with two picnic tables sits on a knoll overlooking Eagle Point. The trail rises another 20 feet to an area of gently rolling fields bursting with golden rod in the fall. This expanse is bordered on the left by red oaks. The trail follows the contours of the field in gradual, but even, ten-foot changes in elevation—the hills resemble a series of swells on the ocean.

Arriving at the intersection of Trail 29 look to the west to see more pockets of oaks scattered across the prairie. The open nature of the this park, coupled with the high number of evergreens, contributes to its charm. Continue past the intersection, and in another 150 yards you get a good view of the northwest end of Eagle Point Lake.

White tail deer abound in the park, indicated by numerous deer tracks on the trail and the lanes of tracks that crisscross the trail. The intersection of Trail 28 is easy to spot because of a prominent landmark rising tall out of the grass: an old windmill from a former homestead. Many of the surrounding meadows are lined in evergreens—a subtle reminder that this land was once farmed. Crops grew in the meadows and the lines of evergreens were planted as windbreaks.

You'll encounter Trail 16 next, a short punch through the thick, wooded area to the right. It appears to lead through a boggy area and across a narrow drainage flowing out of the north end of Eagle Point. If you take this spur it will save you 0.6 mile of walking around another pond and boggy area at the extreme north end of Eagle Point.

However, if you go the extra distance, you'll find it's easy walking! Continue past this shortcut to see more of the pond on the right. This trail follows its oblong shape and loops around its northern end. This area struck me as potentially being very picturesque in the spring. The trail skirts the marshy area to the right before circling back around the top of the loop. More red oaks here, too.

Right at this loop is a knoll of oaks to your left. Check out the ruins of a foundation for some sort of building or dock. At this point on the trail you at the far end of the 3.7-mile loop. A few paces down the trail and 300 yards to the left (beyond the field) is a private residence.

Turn around and catch the lovely vista down the entire length of the pond and Eagle Point Lake beyond. From this point the pond appears to be an elongated S shape. You can see the narrow band of land between Eagle Point and the pond. You can also see the shortcut Trail 16.

This is also near what appears to be the highest point in the park, at least from this vantage point. Open fields spread to the east in long rectangles bordered in more evergreens. This edge of the lake has a lot of deadfall and thick, tangled underbrush. The habitat looks perfect for raccoons, fox, and other critters who use this type of habitat for dens and cover. Deer tracks abound here as well. Continue down the trail, passing by the marker for Trail 15 on your right, the other end of the 0.6-mile shortcut.

The trail turns east, flanked by cottonwoods, dogwoods on the right, and what might have been a wheat field or other planting on the left. A bit farther you'll come upon a small pond on your left and the intersection with Trail 21. Here you'll see a cluster of pin oaks and cedar. Trail 21 leads left to the campground and also connects with other loops. Instead turn right and continue down a short but steep pathway, over a drainage area, and past the intersection with Trail 14, which leads back to the campground (and links up with another trail to the parking lot). If you look over your left shoulder you can catch a glimpse of Lake Elmo.

The last segment of the trail follows along a ridge and is now paralleling the park road about 50 yards through the trees to the left. Any of the next spurs will take you to the main park road and parking area beyond the trailhead.

NEARBY ACTIVITIES

Need more trails? There are several minor loop across the road. Trails 1 and 2 will take you to the south end of Lake Elmo.

#29
Lake Maria State Park

IN BRIEF

The trails that weave through Lake Maria (pronounces Ma-Rye-ah) Park take hikers through many samples of Minnesota's natural history—remnants of the "Big Woods," marshes, and glacier-formed potholes. Noted for its wildlife, including an endangered species of turtle, and a stopping-off point for trumpeter swans, Lake Maria offers a full plate of sights as well as secluded backpacking on winding trails through oak forests.

DIRECTIONS

Take Interstate 94 north to the Monticello exit and County Road 39. Turn north of interstate, then follow signs to left; (CR 39 crosses back over I-94). Follow the road west about 7 miles to CR 11, turn right (north) and go about 1.5 miles. Turn left into the to park entrance, go past the information office, then take your next left. Drive to the trail center at the end of the road.

DESCRIPTION

The trail starts at the western end of the visitor center. This path passes south through a rolling forest of oaks and maples. You immediately get the sense that Lake Maria is a special park. After 0.3 mile you will come to a trail intersection. Continue straight ahead.

As you continue on you will notice that the trail winds its way up and down

KEY AT-A-GLANCE INFORMATION

Length: 3.9 miles

Configuration: A serpentine loop

Difficulty: Easy to moderate; hilly throughout but rises and descents are gradual

Scenery: Very woodsy with many oaks; fabulous in fall

Exposure: Some open areas, most sections under canopy; short section north of road could get hot in full sun

Traffic: Heaviest on southern half except around Bjorkland Lake; eastern edge is less developed, with only trails

Trail Surface: Earthen trails, easily marked, some gravel road surfaces

Hiking Time: 1½–2 hours

Season: All seasons; best in summer and fall

Access: Minnesota State Park fee system—$4 daily, $20 annual permit, $12 handicap/annual permit

Maps: Available at park headquarters at: www.dnr.state.mn.us/parks_and_recreation/state_parks/lake_maria

Special Comments: Popular with students from St. Cloud State College

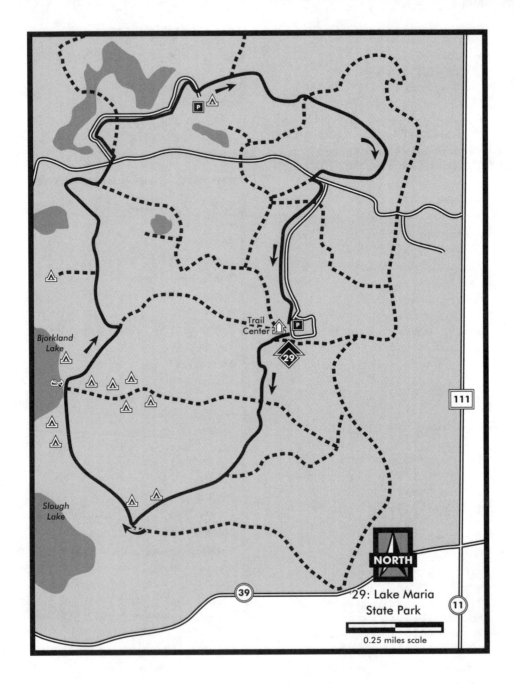

29: Lake Maria
State Park

0.25 miles scale

small hills and knolls—remnants of ages past. These are deposits of the St. Croix glacial moriane formed during the Wisconsin Ice Age. About halfway down, a thick canopy of golden leaves still clings to the trees, even toward the end of fall.

There is little understory along the first sections of this trail, which translates into clear views of this oak forest and the gently rolling terrain. By late fall, the forest floor is a dense, but loose, carpet of oak leaves—a sea of parchment-like leaf patterns you have to literally wade through along the trail. It can be fun walking with the rustling leaves, but be careful, they hide depressions, exposed roots, and the occasional toe-thumping rock—all buried beneath a mantle of golden browns.

As the trail comes up along the top of an oak-covered knoll, Campsite 17, the first of several remote, backpacker campsites in the area, comes into view. Set back into the woods off the main trail, each campsite is a simple cleared area with table and a spot to pitch a tent. Placed about 40 yards apart, campsites are screened by bushes and have a numbered pathways that lead off the main trail.

At this point the hiking trail ends and the horse trail begins. Where the trail Ts, take a right (past Campsite 16) and head north. The trail drops down off the knoll and cuts through a small stand of aspen on this half-mile stretch to the lake. Campsites 14 and 15 are at the bottom of the knoll, just before the trail reaches an open meadow. Beyond the meadow lies Lake Bjorkland. A trailhead at the canoe access point on the lake offers hikers two alternatives: head back to the right through the woods to the visitor center or continue on the horse trail for access to the northern part of the park.

Although I generally prefer not to hike on horse trails, I did decide to continue on this one north from Lake Bjorkland. It's a narrow corridor flanked by oaks. Shortly you will see a hiking trail going straight. Turn left to continue along the horse trail. Soon you will come upon Campsite 7. It sits on a hill overlooking a marshy region below. The trail climbs and dips along this section—more glacial moraine deposits. Elevation varies by about 20 feet in this area. The meandering path climbing up through the oaks really heightens the sense that you are, indeed, embarked on a hike

through the woods. It's this rough, wooded terrain, altered by the terminal moraine topography, that truly adds character to Lake Maria.

A half mile past Campsite 7, you will intersect the park road that connects the entrance to the boat launch and picnic area on Maria Lake about 0.4 mile to the west. If your trek takes you to Maria Lake, set aside some time to enjoy the boardwalk leading to the Zumbrunnen Interpretive Trail. It's about 0.75-mile long, out-and-back, and offers fascinating information on the natural and cultural resources of the area.

Cross this road and head to the entrance to the Primitive Camp Group parking area. Just follow the road past the marshy lake on your left. In these and other spots where the marsh is close to the road be on the look out for a special turtle—one with yellow dots on its back. This is one of the few parks in which you'll see this threatened species in Minnesota. It's called Blanding's turtle.

You'll come to a split in the trail. The left spur goes about 0.3 mile across the marsh to one of two rental camping cabins in the park ($27.50/night, reservations needed). Continue on to the edge of the parking lot where the trail heads back into the woods. A short distance up the trail another spur takes off to the left. It leads to another remote rental cabin, this one on the shore of Putnam Lake on the north boundary of the park. It also takes you to more tent sites at the Putnam Lake backpacking area.

A little over a third of a mile from the last junction, a horse trail cuts through this route. For a side trip you can follow it to the left for a network of loops and other trail segments, including a hike up to Anderson Hill's scenic overlook. Otherwise stay on the main trail, the hiking-only trail, as it works its way along a ridge line.

At what appears to be the highest point along this ridge trail, right as the trial swings back south towards the road, you'll find a bench. Aptly placed, it offers a limited panorama of the wooded ravine at the base of the ridge on the opposite side of the trail. This bench marks the site of a good example of how animals cope in the winter when there is a shortage of food. Look behind the bench at the stand of trees with the dark gray, flaky bark. These are ironwood trees. If you have trouble identifying them, look about 2.5 feet up their trunks from the ground. Notice that the bark has been scraped off. Look closely, those are teeth marks. Check the trees in a 100-foot-diameter circle and you will find this on most of these trees. It is probable that the snow was this deep here, limiting access to veg-etation on the forest floor. Instead animals had to gnaw at the trees available above the snow line, eating the cambium layer beneath the bark. Perhaps deer find ironwood particularly tasty—or they were particularly hungry.

The trail continues around the top of the ravine and then gradually makes its way back to the main park road. You can cross at this point and follow the visitor center road back to the parking lot or continue along the horse trail through the woods. Once you cross the road, its a 0.4-mile hike back to the parking lot and visitor center.

NEARBY ACTIVITIES

Maria Lake connects with Silver Lake for a short but relaxing opportunity to enjoy canoeing.

#30
Lake Minnewashta
Regional Park
(MarshTrail Loop)

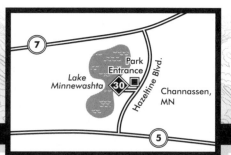

IN BRIEF

The park is but a small corner of a not-so-big lake, yet for shorter hikes that offer moderate changes in elevation and pleasant scenery, it's a good choice for an enjoyable hike. Woods are characteristic oaks, maple, and other hardwoods. The outer-trail loop is trisected for myriad hiking course variables.

DIRECTIONS

From Chanhassen, drive west on County Road 5 past the Minnesota Arboretum. Go right (north) on Hazeltine Boulevard (CR 41) about 1.5 miles to park entrance on left. Upon entering park, turn left and follow the road for about 300 yards to the first picnic area/parking lot on the right. The trailhead is at the far end of the parking lot. Take the trail that follows the lake.

DESCRIPTION

Lake Minnewashta offers two trail systems. The larger system is in the western and southern halves of the park. This is where all the development has taken place. The northern section of the park offers a more primitive setting for hiking.

The Marsh Trail, the object of this hike, is the longest of the three loop sections at Lake Minnewashta. Begin at the parking lot and follow the general shoreline of the lake. No sandy beach here, but there are plenty of the marshy grasses and cattails common to rural lakes

KEY AT-A-GLANCE INFORMATION

Length: 1. 3 miles, with options for shorter loops

Configuration: Balloon

Difficulty: Mostly easy, a few steep hills require moderate effort, but other elevation changes are gradual

Scenery: A pleasant, shallow bay in a woodsy setting

Exposure: The whole trail is shaded

Traffic: Primarily used by those in the immediate residential area

Trail Surface: Narrow; some mowed sections

Hiking Time: 1–1¼ hours

Season: All seasons; summer trails perhaps a little more crowded

Access: $4 daily permit, obtainable through Carver County

Maps: Usually available on site, otherwise through Carver County Parks

Facilities: Developed area of park has rest rooms, drinking water, picnic areas, parking lot

Special Comments: It's like a sampler hiking area—most of the amenities of bigger parks and more diverse terrain

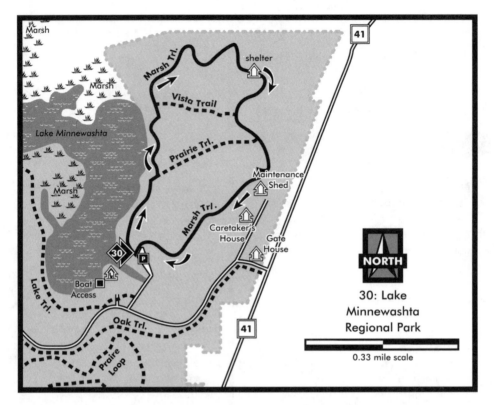

NORTH

30: Lake
Minnewashta
Regional Park

0.33 mile scale

and prairie ponds. If you look straight out across the bay you will see that both entrances to this elongated bay are low, marshy areas.

For about the first 300 yards, the trail is a straight shot through oaks, ash, and maple, as you would expect in this part of Minnesota. As the trail approaches a bay at the northeast end of the lake, look around at all the stately oaks. They are a bit gnarly, but that just adds character to their profile. As you look out over the lake at this point you will be able to see some of the many houses built on the far shore beyond the bay.

The trail climbs about 40 feet above the lake to a ridgeline where you will come to the intersection with the Prairie Trail. The Prairie Trail cuts inland from the lake for about 400 yards and meets up with the Marsh Trail again near

the top of the ridge making a shorter, 0.8-mile loop possible. In the winter this route is popular with cross-country skiers. These trails are clearly marked at trailheads.

Continuing along the main perimeter trail, you are still following the general shoreline of the lake. The trail becomes a little more demanding as it follows the irregular topography. It also continues to ascend as it follows the ridge north. Maples, oaks, even a few black cherry trees are the main trees in these higher reaches on the slopes above the lake. Hiking becomes a bit more moderate as the trail continues to climb to about 80 feet above the lake.

Another 300 yards beyond the Prairie Trail junction is the turn off to Vista Trail. This is the second opportunity to cut across to the other side of the Marsh

Trail. It cuts the distance of the full outer loop by almost one half mile.

At the top of the loop on the Marsh Trail, there are several smaller, earthen paths that lead off of this main trail to the north. Here the trail winds its way through the upland woodlands as it continues to climb slightly along the way. It then starts to turn back down the other side of the loop and head south through more oaks and maples.

Soon you will come upon a shelter on the left. This appears at first to be the high point on the park trail, but that's still ahead. On rivers they call a false headland on the shore "Point No Point." This part of the trail could be called "Top No Top" because it soon becomes apparent that there is still a little more uphill hiking to do. However, there is a bench and drinking water here so it's a good place to stop.

It's about another 400 yards to the junction with the upper Vista Trail. After this, it's less than 300 yards to the Prairie Trail junction on the right. The highest point in the park (as best as I could determine from the faint topo lines on the map) is about 200 yards past the Prairie Trail. Here you come upon a small, but welcome, stand of white pines.

The trail appears to climb slightly beyond this point. There is a maintenance shed about 100 yards past what the map shows as the highest contour line (1000') in the park. Another 300 yards and the Caretakers House is off to the left.

The trail reaches an open meadow— one of those oak prairie areas. Ash trees are scattered throughout this section. There is a small stand of cedar trees that are in contrast with the others. This immediately catches one's eye coming out of the woods. I would expect this meadow to be blooming wildly with wildflowers throughout spring and summer.

At this point the trail is about 150 yards off and parallel to the road that goes to the Caretaker's House as it heads into a patch of trees and dense understory dominated by elderberry and buckthorns. The trail drops down through this island of trees and shrubs on its way back to the parking lot at the bottom.

NEARBY ACTIVITIES

The Minnesota Arboretum is only a few miles away. Its a living showcase of Minnesota flora. There are hiking trails throughout its grounds, too.

#31
Lake Nokomis

IN BRIEF

The most prominent and popular lake in South Minneapolis, Nokomis is situated right on the Grand Rounds Trail on the leg of Minnehaha Creek just west of the Falls. This lake typifies the lakes throughout Minneapolis and St. Paul that are popular courses for hikers of all ages and abilities. Besides its paved walkways and spacious grassy areas, Nokomis offers hikers a tree-lined promenade along most of its shoreline. Several areas are reverting back to more natural states, providing hikers with a hint what wilder lakes are like outside the limits of the city.

DIRECTIONS

Take Cedar Avenue south to Minnehaha Parkway. Continue east (turning left) to the Lake Nokomis Parkway entrance (signed). Turn right, go about 200 yards to the parking lot. You can also turn left at the stoplight just before Cedar Avenue Bridge. Turn left and follow the parkway about a quarter mile to the concession area and swimming beach.

DESCRIPTION

Of all the lakes in the Grand Round loop, my favorite is Lake Nokomis. It's the lake I grew up around, paddled my canoes and kayaks, and fished with my great grandfather from England. We always told people we "lived near Lake Nokomis." I've walked around this lake

KEY AT-A-GLANCE INFORMATION

Length: 2.75 miles

Configuration: An oblong circle that closely follows the shoreline of the lake

Difficulty: Very easy; wheelchair accessible, although pavement is uneven in places

Scenery: Groomed lawns with open, tree-lined views of the lake

Exposure: Mostly full sun, some shade

Traffic: Very popular lake for South Minneapolitans, but plenty of room for all

Trail Surface: Concrete sidewalk or blacktop in some areas; older sections can be uneven

Hiking Time: 1–1.5 hours

Season: All seasons; trails maintained year-round

Access: Free; plenty of parking around perimeter of lake parkway

Maps: None with specific detail; all city maps will show location

Facilities: Main beach has concession stand, bathhouse, rest rooms, drinking water, picnic tables; outhouses at secondary beach

Special Comments: This is the kind of lake walk you can do over and over

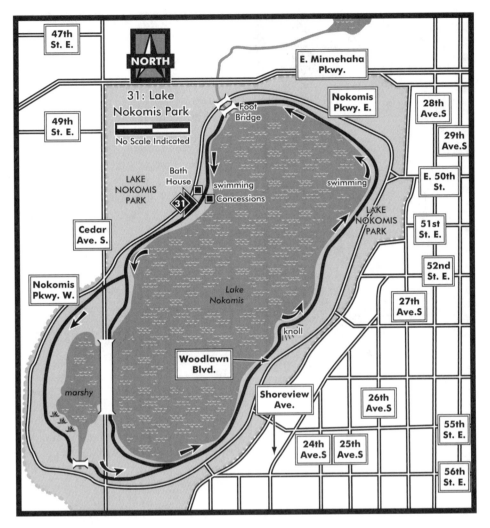

during a winter storm at 30° below 0 and in sweltering 100° summer heat.

As with all the city lakes, you can start and end your hike anywhere along its pathway. I like to start along the boulevard—at one of the many turn-out parking areas provided. For this hike, however, start at the concession stand parking area. It's near the beach and refreshments are available throughout the summer.

Head south along the wide walkway past the canoe racks and the boat access ramp. Several years ago Lake Nokomis was devastated by a wind storm that literally tore mature trees out of the ground by their roots. Some survived, but with good portions of their crowns lost to the wind shears, and some of the trees in this section bear those scars. The path doesn't closely follow the willows growing along the shoreline. Stop anywhere along the path to enjoy the great vistas of the lake.

At Cedar Avenue you have a choice: continue around the outside edge of the lake (and the part you'll bypass if you cross over the Cedar Avenue Bridge) or

111

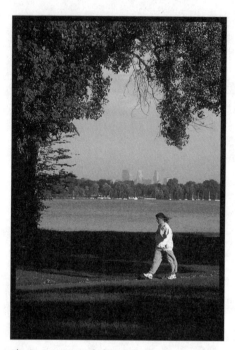

The Twin Cities' Skyline seen beyond Lake Nokomis.

the bridge to stop and enjoy the sights. Even though its not an especially big lake, Nokomis does get its share of sailboats and other watercraft—all of which add to the view of the lake from the bridge.

After the bridge, the pathway continues around the southern end of the lake. It closely follows the shoreline and meanders among the massive trunks and buttresses of giant cottonwoods. There were some majestic trees in this area before the big blow-down. Large, eight-foot-diameter stump bases are all that remain of these gigantic lakeside trees. As you continue, you will start to see the beautiful island of skyscrapers in downtown Minneapolis poking their heads over the trees beyond the far side of the lake. There are several places along this shoreline where you can frame some lovely shots of downtown's crown.

About 0.75 mile after crossing the bridge, and half way up the east side of the lake, there is a slight rise in the trail to a small knoll. A drinking fountain and the start of a Vita-Course (a series of fitness stations along the route with a variety of exercises you can do) makes this a popular gathering spot for walkers.

Continuing north, the area around the trail opens onto a long, grassy area and open shorelines along the lake. A bit farther and you will come upon the swimming beach. It, too, is a gathering point and offers the only rest rooms (portables) on this side of the lake. This beach is at the bottom of the hill of the 50th Street access to the Nokomis parkway. A couple of blocks up the hill and you'll find a little business corner with groceries and a sidewalk café. I think there is an ice cream shop there, too.

The path continues around the north end of the lake. There is a section of

take the bridge for a loftier view of both sections of the lake. If you are into a quiet, less-traveled walk, cross Cedar and continue on the path. It leads through open, grassy areas and cuts back closer to the lake after following the edge of a wetlands area. It then goes into a stand of cottonwoods and other lowland vegetation that lines a small feeder creek for Lake Nokomis on the extreme southwest corner of the lake. This is not a maintained area, far from it at times, but it is a place to see some turtles and song birds. It brings hikers back to Cedar Avenue beyond the southern end of the bridge for a reconnection with the main lake pathway a few hundred yards after crossing the street.

If you decide to take the bridge, you have the traffic noise to contend with, but also the expansive view of the lake. There is even a turn-out platform on cedar trees covering a small area where an outflow feeding Minnehaha Creek flows by just beyond the northern tip of Lake Nokomis. A small, arching footbridge crosses the outlet and continues to wind a bit through more cedars and spruce. The walkway continues through the swimming beach area and past the concession stand to repeat its course around the lake.

NEARBY ACTIVITIES

You can follow the Minnehaha Creek Parkway east to the Falls, or back along the creek as it meanders through south Minneapolis. Eventually, about 3 miles to the west, you can walk around Lake Harriet, Lake Calhoun, Lake of the Isles, and Cedar Lake. The first three are described elsewhere in this book as the City Lakes Trail.

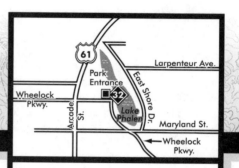

#32
Lake Phalen

IN BRIEF

Well-known to Twin Cities residents as a popular golf course and urban lake, the Phalen-Keller area provides hiking opportunities for residents and visitors alike. Typical of a city park-and-lake system, Phalen offers a full menu of activities from picnic area to swimming beach to the Lakeside Activities Center. The lake offers a sense of openness in the middle of developed neighborhoods.

DIRECTIONS

From Minneapolis, take Interstate 94 into downtown St. Paul. Then take I-35 to Larpenteur Avenue, exit to the east (right) about 1.5 miles, and intersect the park at the golf course. You can also turn south from Larpenteur until you meet Wheelock Parkway, a meandering road only a few blocks south of Larpenteur. Turn left, heading east again and go about 1.5 miles to the park entrance. From St. Paul, Phalen Park is intersected by Larpenteur Avenue on the east side and Johnson Parkway from the south (go north off of I-94). To access to the park from the west, follow the directions from Minneapolis.

DESCRIPTION

The Phalen Park area of eastern St. Paul has been attracting visitors for years with the combined attractions of Lake Phalen and Keller Golf Course. The park and golf course are situated in the middle of

KEY AT-A-GLANCE INFORMATION

Length: 3.2 miles, with 0.8-mile loop option

Configuration: One full circle with extended spur if desired

Difficulty: Easy; paved, smooth paths, level throughout along lake's shoreline

Scenery: Pleasantly groomed and landscaped, typical of many city lakes and parks

Exposure: Mostly full sun, some shade

Traffic: Light, but popular for leisurely walks throughout the week

Trail Surface: Completely paved

Hiking Time: 1–1½ hours

Season: All seasons; walkway cleared in winter

Access: Parking within park, along turn-outs, no fees

Maps: Not readily available at park; online at www.stpaul.gov/depts/parks/

Facilities: Fully developed park with playground, picnic area with pavilion and BBQ grills, full-service bath house, rest rooms, drinking water

Special Comments: One of several larger lakes in the eastern half of St. Paul—quite popular

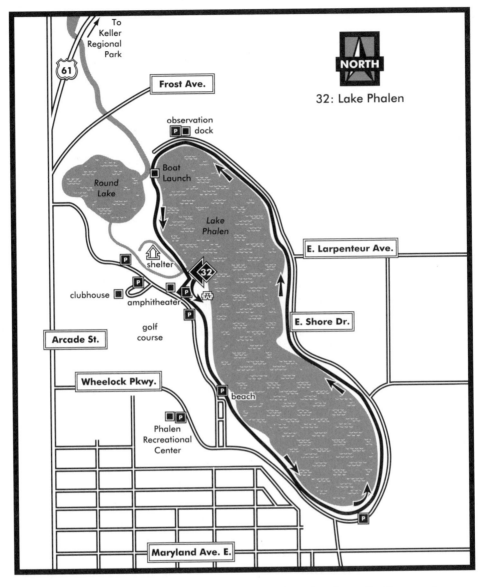

solid residential neighborhoods. The open lake and easy access to its trail make it a popular getaway from the compactness of the city that surrounds it.

All the development around the park is situated on the western shores of Lake Phalen. Ample parking allows hikers to start from several spots along this end of the lake. Start at the picnic pavilion at the northwest end of the lake. The shoreline is steep here but the trail will soon take you down next to the water. Head south along the paved pathway past the Lakeside Center. This is only 0.1 mile from the picnic area and has its own parking lot. A nice stand of oaks separates the two areas while providing a somewhat lofty view of the lake from atop the embankment.

The trail continues along the lake but leaves the shoreline for about 0.3 mile as it winds up and along a knoll between the Lakeside Center and the beach area. This knoll has a scattered planting of oaks and Scotch pine. Once you pass the swimming beach you are near the lake's edge.

The path follows the lake for some distance while it parallels Wheelock Parkway. The lake is always in view at this point and this enables you to look to the far northern shore from anywhere along this entire stretch. Willows and cottonwoods, typically moist region/lowland trees, line the lake in this area. The path follows the lake for 0.7–0.8 mile before swinging east. There is a huge willow tree there with a diameter of over five feet. Imagine an entire embankment covered with these monsters!

At 1 mile, you'll come to another parking area. This is an alternate starting point if you don't want to actually go into the park near the beach and picnic areas. Beyond this parking lot, you'll see more varieties of trees—pin oaks and locust—and varied landscaped species planted to offer diversity and some shade. Along this stretch of the lake, the path is about four feet from the water's edge at the top of a gradual embankment.

By 1.5 miles the residential neighborhood is fairly close to the trail, separated only by East Shore Drive Boulevard. Birch trees have been added to the pin oaks around the area. This is only 0.2 mile from a few benches and another knoll where the trail forks. Hikers can continue left along the lake, while bikers must go up the knoll and to the right for about 0.2 mile before rejoining the trail along the lake again.

At 2.5 miles the trail cuts back to the west at the northern end of the lake. There is yet another parking lot and an observation platform. In the winter, this area remains open for the visiting geese and ducks that pass through the area. It is also at a junction of trails that lead into Keller Park and the Keller Picnic Area.

If you go to the right beyond the platform, you'll link up with a short trail system that winds through the outflow area of Keller Lake, adding about 0.8 mile to the hike. It is a primitive area compared to the shoreline of Phalen. It's marshy with more natural stands of trees. There is a small bridge across the creek that goes a short distance to the western edge of the park boundary. It also takes you to the southern edge of Phalen Golf Course. That trail also links up with a trail that goes around Round Lake, a small knob of water connected to Phalen at the mouth of a creek flowing into Phalen from the north. This path leads back to the picnic area where the hike started.

If you take a left immediately after the observation deck, you'll come to a footbridge over this same feeder creek. This stretch of the hike is about 0.4 mile long and takes you back to the picnic pavilion.

NEARBY ACTIVITIES

Phalen Lake is surrounded by residential neighborhoods to the south, Keller Golf Course to the west, and access to the Gateway Trail to the north. The Gateway Trail is a great hiking/biking path that cuts a swath through St. Paul. Bring your clubs and/or your bicycle for extended options at Phalen.

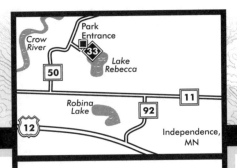

#33
Lake Rebecca

Crow River

Park Entrance

Lake Rebecca

50

Robina Lake

92

11

12

Independence, MN

IN BRIEF

An expansive park with good examples of how a forest slowly regains the abandoned agricultural fields of early settlers. The trail circles Lake Rebecca through meadows and younger-growth forests.

DIRECTIONS

Drive west from Minneapolis on US Highway 12 past Maple Plain towards Delano. Just before Delano turn right (north) on County Road 92 and drive about 2 miles to CR 11. Turn left (west) and go 2.5 miles to CR 50 (Town Line Road). Turn right (north) and drive 1.5 miles to the park. Upon entering the park, take a left and go to the far end of the parking lot. The trailhead begins at the extreme north end of the lot.

DESCRIPTION

Geologically speaking, Lake Rebecca Park Reserve lies on the ground moraine deposited by the Des Moines lobe of the Wisconsin Ice Age glacial material. The park has rolling countryside that had been clear-cut by early settlers for agricultural use. Much of that land continues to revert naturally back to a "big woods" forested type in what is called "old field" succession. Maple and basswood forests are slowly regaining footholds as this park returns to a more woodsy nature. The Hennepin Regional Park District is still acquiring land for the park. When complete, Lake Rebecca

KEY AT-A-GLANCE INFORMATION

Length: 6.5 miles

Configuration: Loop

Difficulty: Easy; gentle rises/falls in elevation with no strenuous inclines

Scenery: Woodsy and advanced meadows, few vistas of the lake

Exposure: Mostly full sun, some shade

Traffic: Shared with bicycles, light pedestrian traffic

Trail Surface: Paved throughout

Hiking Time: 2¼–3 hours

Season: Trails closed November 1 through March 31

Access: $5 daily vehicle permit, $27 Patrons Annual Hennepin Parks permit

Maps: Available at park headquarters, or at www.hennepinparks.org

Facilities: Picnic area with shelter, concessions, rest rooms

Special Comments: Plan time to visit the Trumpeter Swan Restoration Project area

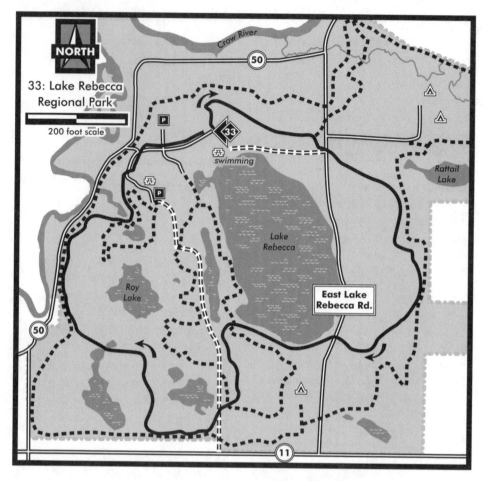

33: Lake Rebecca
Regional Park

200 foot scale

50

Crow River

33

swimming

P

P

Roy
Lake

Lake
Rebecca

Rattail
Lake

East Lake
Rebecca Rd.

50

11

will comprise over 2,500 acres. The bike/hike trail offers the best all-around experience at Lake Rebecca.

Head north on the paved trail, where you'll see box elders and open, grassy, rolling hills giving way to overgrown prairie-like country as the trail meanders through some of the higher elevations in the park. Soon, however, the trail drops into a thicket of maples and basswoods as it continues along a ridge that seems to follow an old river channel. The Crow River is a few hundred yards to your left, but the trail never approaches the river.

You'll come to a short section of split rail fencing on the left and a subtle over-look onto a small pothole partially visible

through the thick understory. Continue along the ridge, which is about 25 feet above the forest floor on your left. The trail then doglegs slightly to the left before continuing on about 0.7 mile to its intersection with Lake Rebecca Road.

However, just before the road, there will be a clearly-marked fork in the trail. Take the right fork (the left takes you to Lake Sarah, 0.5 mile to the north) which will take you towards Lake Rebecca and the interior of the park. You will come up and out of the thicket-like forest area onto a hilly, meadow-like area with sumac, box elder, and a few scattered cedars. The gravel road intersects the trail just as you come out onto this opening.

Like others in the park, this meadow represents one of the many stages of recovery the park's open areas are making as they slowly return to the forested cover that existed prior to the settlers' presence 150 years ago. You will notice taller trees already making a stand in this meadow. Farther along the hike, meadows in varying stages of regrowth can be compared to each other as this rejuvenation process continues.

The trail slowly climbs for about a half mile to the top of the meadow. At the very top of the climb, check out the elm-like trees on your left. These are ironwood. They tend to be tall and slender and their leaves are very much like elm leaves except they are thinner and finer. You will also find sumac, burr oak, ash, and dogwood—all examples of the types of vegetation slowly encroaching onto the prairie areas.

The trail cuts through a thicket of sumac before dropping down as it meanders along the eastern section of the lake. At about 1.5 miles you'll come upon a picnic table and the trail will cross over a creek running from Rattail Lake to the east. The trail carves a few big **S** turns then starts to rise again through a growth of ironwood and a mix of mature maples, burr oaks, and box elder—all in a thick understory.

Soon the trail opens back up to a corridor, a more airy canopy of shorter trees on each side. At about 2.3 miles this trail again crosses Lake Rebecca Road and drops into stands of maples. As you come out onto marshy lowlands at the southern end of Lake Rebecca, the trail again cuts through more forested areas of box elder and maples.

The trail follows the south end of the lake for about a half mile. Cattails, rushes, and willows are the dominant vegetation in this area—all typical of a Minnesota marsh. At about 3 miles the trail cuts sharply to the left and away from the lake. You cross an intersection with the bike trail and a spur to the group camp. Stay on the main trail and as it turns look over your right shoulder and you'll see a small, hidden bay of Lake Rebecca. This is a good birding area for waterfowl, perhaps even a crane or great blue heron.

From here the trail climbs up from the lake into another meadow area. Again, check out the encroachment of taller vegetation and trees into this grassland. You'll see saplings of ash and aspen whips mixed with other advancing species. You'll also notice a plantation-like row of trees on the rolling hills above the lake.

The trail drops down to lower elevations once more as it parallels the horse trail along the southern boundary of the park. It climbs again through maples, ironwoods—larger trees than the last section—and swings north for about a half mile before turning west.

At about 4.1 miles the trail enters a meadow area, this one with several winding hills and great expanses of open spaces. The trail turns west for about 0.4 mile. At about 4.7 miles along the trail there is another picnic table along the edge of yet another marshy area. There is a small parking lot/staging area for the horse trail on the left at about 4.9 miles.

The trail once more heads north, this time following the western boundary of the park. At about 6 miles the trail reconnects with the park road and it's about 0.5 mile back to the parking lot.

NEARBY ACTIVITIES

Immediately accessible is the short, "hiking only" loop to the right of the main entrance. It's only 0.5-mile long through a forested area within the park. You are also close to Lake Sarah Park and its recreational amenities

#34
Lawrence Trail, Minnesota Valley

IN BRIEF

A few miles south of Louisville Swamp, the Lawrence section offers more views of the lowland floodplain with trails tied into the upland hardwood forests that line this river in eastern Minnesota.

DIRECTIONS

From Minneapolis, head south on US Highway 169 past Shakopee to Jordan. Turn right (north) onto County Road 9 for 0.1 mile to CR 57 (190th Street West). Turn left and go about 4 miles to the park's Trail Center entrance on right. Park in front of Trail Center building.

DESCRIPTION

There is hardly a stretch of the Minnesota River that hasn't been hiked since humans first set foot along its shores. Clearly, each of the segments designated for recreation along the corridor that comprises the Minnesota Valley State Recreation Area has ample trails and paths along which hikers can roam.

Follow the gravel road into the park entrance marked Trail Center and go to the right to the end of the parking lot. A path leads to the left of the Trail Center building and immediately forks. You want to take the right fork designated as the Hiking Club Trail. The left fork is a horse trail that can be quite muddy even in the middle of summer. Save it for an additional hike option on a dry afternoon.

KEY AT-A-GLANCE INFORMATION

Length: 4.8 miles

Configuration: Balloon

Difficulty: Easy; level throughout but sections could be excessively muddy or flooded in the spring

Scenery: Lowland; river bottoms on one side, upper hardwood forest growth on the other

Exposure: Intermittent sun and shade throughout hike

Traffic: Popular with equestrians (on separate trails); not known by many

Trail Surface: Mowed grass, some hard-pack earthen trails, soft and muddy in lower sections, particularly in spring or after heavy rains

Hiking Time: 1½–2½ hours

Season: All seasons; sections may be impassable in early spring due to rainfall

Access: No fees

Maps: Available at Park Ranger Office

Facilities: Boat and canoe ramps, camping, picnic area, trail center shelter

Special Comments: Wear waterproof high boots if planning on hiking any of the horse trails along the river

120

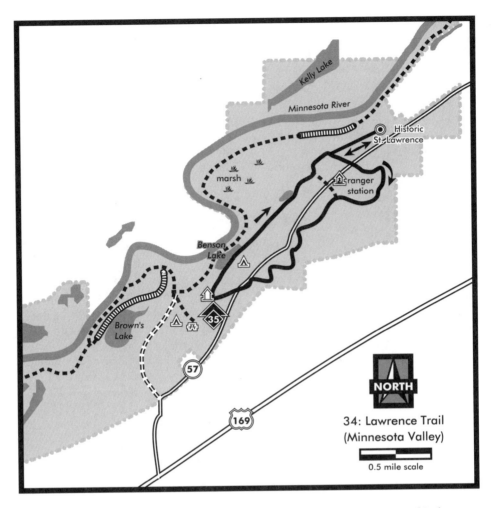

The right fork leads through a wooded area dominated at first by elms and then by the mix of species common to this part of the state: ash, box elder, and oaks. Within 0.2 mile you will see Beason Lake on your left. More backwater slough than pond, Beason extends for 0.6 mile as it parallels this trail.

Along the way you'll pass spur trails to the left that head back toward the road and the campground to the southeast. A bench has been placed at an opening in the vegetation growing up along the lake for a restful view across the narrow waterway and to the woods on the left.

This section is heavily covered in box elders, a common lowland tree. Likewise, silver maples sprout like weeds along the trail.

You'll come to a gravel road that leads to the right, but don't take it; stay on the main trail. Soon you'll come to another open view of the marsh. At this point you can see beyond the lake toward the vast expanse of marsh that spreads from the trail toward the banks of the Minnesota River just beyond the distant row of trees. The horse trail you could have taken at the fork at the start of this trail winds through those trees along the river.

Just past a noticeable low drainage area you'll see many smaller boulders embedded in the forest floor and along the trail. Off to the left is a huge boulder about the size of a washing machine. How do you suppose it got there? Imagine a glacier carrying such rocks around like grains of sand until they settled into the ground as the glacier receded.

That would have been the scene over 10,000 years ago as the glacial River Warren flowed through this area. It was a drainage system from the great glacial Lake Agassiz to the west. River Warren is responsible for cutting the huge valley through which the Minnesota River runs today. That valley is over 5 miles wide in some spots and nearly 300 feet deep.

Continuing down the trail another 0.1 mile you will come to a meadow on the right. At the far end stands a stone house typical of those built in the nineteenth century. You'll have a chance to learn more about the history of the area farther up the trail, so continue on.

The trail now cuts across a willow-lined causeway over a wet drainage area. At the culvert you are right at water's edge of the large marsh to the left (west). This will be a good viewing area for waterfowl, particularly during the spring migration.

Immediately past the drainage area the trail passes through a stand of box elder and ironwood trees. You then come to a spur on the right that leads back to the road at the Ranger Station. Stay to the left and continue on for another 0.3 mile until you reach the next trail intersection. You have a major trail choice to make here.

You can continue straight ahead and quickly reach an intersection with the gravel road. This cuts out 1.2 miles of hiking, but you will miss an interesting interpretive site. If you wish to visit the site, as this description does, turn left and walk 0.6 mile until you come to the park's official historic site, the Samuel B. Strait homestead. Built in 1857 and restored in 2000, the house is the remaining symbol of the Strait's 1,000-acre homestead settled in 1855. This and other homes were part of a town site that anticipated prosperity from the railroad that was to pass through the area. The railroad did work its way through the area, but it never developed into a stop—and the town never blossomed.

After exploring the house, you can choose to return along the spur trail, or follow the trail out to the gravel park road near the southeast park boundary, turning right at the intersection with the gravel road and hiking back to the next trail intersection. There you'll turn left (away from the river) to continue the hike. Either backtracking or continuing on past the house, both trails meet back up at the same trail intersection with the park roadway.

You are now on a series of lobes that wind back-and-forth along the wooded "high country" of the park between the gravel road and the park's boundary. This first lobe is 0.9 mile and meanders through stands of gnarly burr oaks, ash, basswood—typical of upland woods. The first intersection on the right will be a spur heading to the Ranger Station at the road. Continue straight, past the intersection, and onto the second lobe. This is a 1.4-mile section that continues to wind through upland forest. There's not a lot of changes in vegetation as the mowed, wide pathway gracefully winds through the trees.

There is one section about half way along this lobe that I found particularly appealing. You'll come upon a small stand of tall-and-narrow aspens, their powdery white-gray bark almost glowing in the sunlight. These are thin, straight trees with heart-shaped leaves, a total contrast to the gnarly burr oak immediately behind them. Slightly taller, but much wider, the multi-lobed, dark green leaves of the stately oak with its twisting branches are totally opposite to the modest aspen. Together they form an appealing contrast along the trail's edge.

The trail crosses a wet area via a wooden, planked walkway just before turning very closely toward the road. On the left you'll pass a wet, marshy area thick with rushes (Torrey's Rush) a common plant that grows very densely in this kind of marsh. Another wooden pathway, this one about 50 feet long, takes you over another excessively moist part of the trail.

At the end of the 1.4-mile lobe, a spur trail shoots off to the right. This heads back across the road and to the entrance of the Quarry Campground, the main camping area for this park.

The last lobe takes the trail back across the road and diagonally through the woods as it leads back to the parking lot for the last 0.4 mile of the hike. You re-enter the parking lot on the right side of the Trail Center building.

NEARBY ACTIVITIES

Just north of Jordan is the Louisville Swamp section of the Minnesota Valley State Recreation Area. Excellent hiking and historical landmarks (see page 133).

#35
Lebanon Hills Regional Park (Holland/Jensen Lakes Loop)

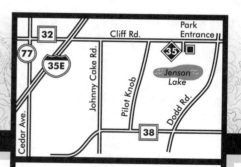

IN BRIEF

Located in the heart of the suburbs south of Minneapolis, Lebanon Hills is one of the more diverse parks in the Dakota County system. There are more than a dozen lakes scattered throughout rolling hills with clusters of oaks and maples and open pockets of meadows and marshes. One of the prettiest lakes in the region—unnamed no less—greets hikers deep within the park.

DIRECTIONS

From Minneapolis, drive south on Cedar Avenue/Minnesota Highway 77 to Cliff Road (Exit 4A). From St. Paul, drive south on Interstate 35 East to Cliff Road (Exit 93); turn left (east) and drive past Pilot Knob Road to theHolland Lake entrance on the right. The trailhead is at the parking lot's far right corner.

DESCRIPTION

Like so many other suburban parks that sit literally in the middle of residential suburban sprawl, Lebanon Hills quickly lures the visitor into the heart of the park and away from any reminders of that fringe of development. The Holland-Jensen Lake Trail leads the hiker away from the big houses skirting the boundary of the park and into hilly terrain covered in oaks and meadows, sprinkled with ponds and lakes.

Dropping down from the parking lot, take the spur trail leading hikers along

KEY AT-A-GLANCE INFORMATION

Length: 2.6 miles

Configuration: Balloon

Difficulty: Easy to moderate with numerous small changes in elevation

Scenery: Peaceful and picturesque from rolling hills to quiet lakes

Exposure: Wooded, shady areas are evenly mixed with open, exposed meadows

Traffic: Very popular, particularly with joggers

Trail Surface: Wide, compacted grass trails, some earthen paths

Hiking Time: 1½ hours

Season: All seasons; allows hunting briefly in fall; many trails open for cross-country skiing

Access: $5 daily vehicle permit, $27 Patrons Annual Hennepin Parks permit

Maps: Dakota County Parks Map or online at www.co.dakota.mn.us/parks/hills

Facilities: Parking, picnic shelter, swimming beach, playground, canoe trail, rest rooms at trailhead, campground, potable water nearby

Special Comments: Surrounded by townhouses, strip malls, and freeways, this park sees heavy use yet maintains its country character

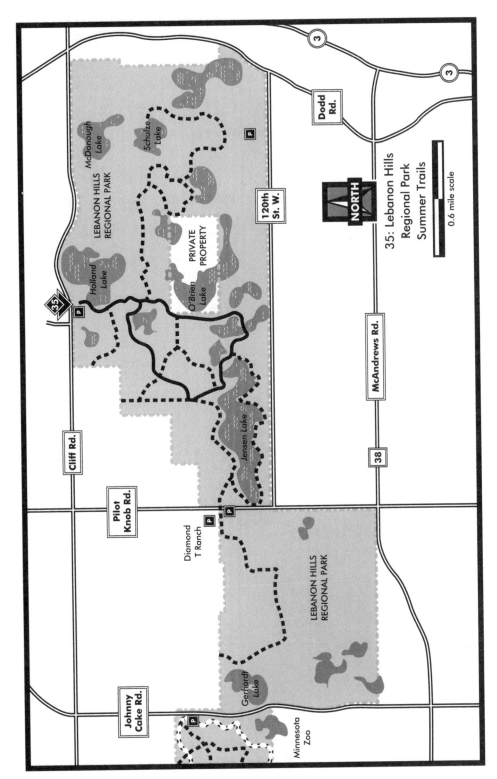

35: Lebanon Hills
Regional Park
Summer Trails

NORTH

0.6 mile scale

LEBANON HILLS REGIONAL PARK

McDonough Lake

Schulze Lake

Holland Lake

O'Brien Lake

PRIVATE PROPERTY

Jensen Lake

120th St. W.

Dodd Rd.

Cliff Rd.

Pilot Knob Rd.

Johnny Cake Rd.

Diamond T Ranch

Gerhardt Lake

LEBANON HILLS REGIONAL PARK

Minnesota Zoo

McAndrews Rd.

38

35

3

3

125

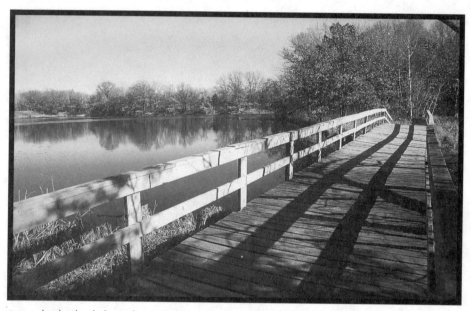

A wooden bridge links trails at Lebanon Hills Regional Park.

the west side of Holland Lake toward a network of trails that allow one to select several loop options. Most will lead back to this short, quarter-mile segment and a short, repeated journey up this same trail spur. In the spring, or after a good rain, expect this first section around Holland Lake to be a bit wet. The trail winds through a fairly thick growth of aspen, birch, wild cherry, and buckthorn before encountering one of the many hills of Lebanon. Continuing through a stand of aspen, the trail soon leads hikers to an open meadow and the first of many trail intersections (all fairly well marked, but get a map at the trailhead parking lot). Each map trail marker has a "you are here" indicator that corresponds to the trail map. Continue straight ahead.

Less than a quarter mile into the park, this trail is winding its way through several species of oak that border a meadow at the southwest end of the lake. Out of the woods south of Holland Lake the country is a series of gently rolling hills. The trail is lined with sumac and young

oaks pop up intermittently across the grassy fields. I was here in late fall but would expect to see a spring profusion of wildflowers common to the upland meadows of central Minnesota.

Numerous ponds, all nameless, pocket the area's recesses adding to a pleasant country setting of rolling countryside, islands of hardwood trees, and a patchwork quilt of prairie-like meadows.

Hike past another trail on your left and as you approach the northwest corner of O'Brien Lake and you'll come upon a covered picnic table and your first good glimpse of O'Brien. Stay on the trails here because most of the property around this lake is private.

The trails are shared with joggers. The wide pathway and gently undulating terrain probably provides a good workout for runners—as it does for faster-paced hikers. After a good snowfall, expect to see cross-country skiers as well.

Continuing south along the western edge of the lake, the trail becomes wide and rutted—more road than trail. Just past the table and a trail junction, about 200 yards farther south, a nesting platform for ospreys and other raptors has been erected on the left. It sits atop a tall pole. Approach it slowly and quietly and you may be rewarded with a glimpse of local raptor residents.

Few sections of this trail maintain any one characteristic for very long. This rutted roadway soon opens onto yet another meadow with a surface that appears to have been scoured by a ground fire recently. This provides a good field demonstration on the positive benefits of brush fires, especially if one knew what was growing here before and what successions occur as new growth emerges.

There are several horse trails intertwined throughout this entire park. Intersections with the hiking trail are common. Personally, I try to stay away from the trails that shared usage. Horse trails get ground into a very deep yet fine dust that can be tiring to walk on for any distance. Also, I have yet to experience a quiet walk when riders are present. I guess horseback riding and talking loud go hand in hand. These trails are pretty obvious, but are usually marked as well.

A little over a mile along this trail on the right is a beautiful country lake surrounded by oaks and birch that blanket the steep banks of this watery gem. I imagine it's beautiful in the summer because it is absolutely gorgeous in the fall. Golds and oranges and reds are speckled throughout the trees that line its banks. A shallow bay on the far side creates an opening in the shoreline, and the marshy area beyond adds a smattering of cattails to the scene. This unnamed lake is on the Jensen Lake chain that enables canoeists to see this park from yet another perspective.

The trail cuts deeply into the steep banks along the southeastern edge of the

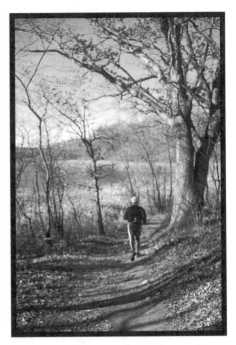

A jogger on Lebanon Hills' earthen trails.

lake. You can stop anywhere along this side of the lake to get peaceful views of the far side. Stately birch trees line the southern shoreline. This lake feeds into yet another at the extreme southern end. A picturesque footbridge provides a dry crossing and a dual vantage point for looking back over the first lake or southeast along the canoe route. Just before the footbridge, a small knoll with a picnic table provides a handy resting place for hikers and paddlers alike.

The pathway becomes more serpentine as it continues north around the western edge of this lake. Oak trees line the pockets of clearings to the west.

Less than a quarter mile farther, Jensen Lake comes into view. There are several trail intersections that offer options should you want to extend your hike. The first one to the left (south) takes hikers around the southern end of Jensen Lake to another **T** junction. From there hikers can either continue around the entire lake to the right (for an additional 2.2 miles) or cut back to the left and towards the other parking lot and playground area.

This hike stays to the right and continues along the northern shore, then loops back toward Holland Lake. You'll notice Jensen Lake's western and northern shores are developed and there are quite a few houses. This route, too, leads past some development but it will eventually get you back to the hiking trails or a short segment of one of the horse trails. This area seems especially alive with birds. Expect to see quite a few varieties in the summer. In late fall, chickadees, downy woodpeckers, and scores of cedar waxwings dominated a small section of woods just north of the trail junction that leads away from the lake.

Shortly after leaving the lake, the narrow trail intersects a road. To the right is a private residence; to the left the road leads to another parking area. There is a narrow pathway straight ahead across the road heading up through the understory. Take this trail. It breaks out onto a wider horse trail (the spot you'd end up if you looped around Jensen Lake). Taking the horse path enables you to make a loop back to the spur leading to the parking lot without a lot of backtracking.

This stretch of the trail is quite sandy in places. It's easier to walk on the edges of such trails—and probably safer. This wide section goes for about a third of a mile through mature stands of oaks. The area is more consistently hilly than other areas of the park. It takes you back along the opposite side of the picturesque but nameless lake encountered earlier. The trail then cuts back into the woods. Eventually you'll return to the spur that led you down from the parking lot. As you come to the end of the lake remember to take the second trail, not the first. The second one, about 30–40 yards farther—is the correct one. It climbs back up to the park entrance where the trailhead started.

A word of caution: If you are planning a hike through Lebanon Hills in the fall, check the posted signs explaining the limited deer hunting that is allowed in this park. Typically these hunting times are restricted to a few short periods during the week, from early morning until noon.

NEARBY ACTIVITIES

The Minnesota Zoo, literally a few blocks away, has paved trails tying all the outside viewing areas together. Also at the zoo is the Omni Theatre—expect great programming throughout the year.

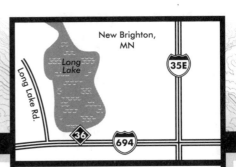

#36
Long Lake

IN BRIEF

Short on distance and limited on scenery, the trail does offer a pleasant hike along a lake and through a historic corridor of nineteenth century commerce.

DIRECTIONS

From St. Paul, take Interstate 35 East north to I-694. Go west on I-694 to Long Lake Road (Exit 40) and exit right. Turn right immediately on top of the exit ramp into the park. Park at the lake's southern tip at the end of the road.

DESCRIPTION

While you probably won't even have to pack a water bottle for this hike, it does offer a respite from the urban bustle that surrounds it. Located literally an exit ramp off of the Twin Cities' very busy I-694 and flanked by equally trafficked I-35 East, Long Lake's hiking trail takes a short course through the neighborhood's municipal history while skirting a modest but activity-rewarding lake.

The trailhead is at the far end of the parking lot, near the rest rooms. You shouldn't get lost on these ten-foot-wide, paved trails that always have the lake on their left (on the way up). The first 0.4 mile passes through a stately and mature mixed stand of box elder, oak, and cottonwoods. The trail cuts through these trees and then is flanked by them on the shore side of the trail. The entire

KEY AT-A-GLANCE INFORMATION

Length: 1.85 miles

Configuration: Balloon

Difficulty: One long, gradual incline at top of loop, but otherwise easy

Scenery: Pleasantly "woodsy" with rolling hills, southern exposure to lake, and marsh country

Exposure: Mostly full sun, some shade

Traffic: Popular as neighborhood park, especially on evenings and weekends

Trail Surface: Paved

Hiking Time: 1 hour

Season: All seasons

Access: No fees

Maps: Available from Ramsey County or at www.co.ramsey.mn.us/Parks/maps/long_with_legend2

Special Comments: One of few open-space parks in this area north of St. Paul

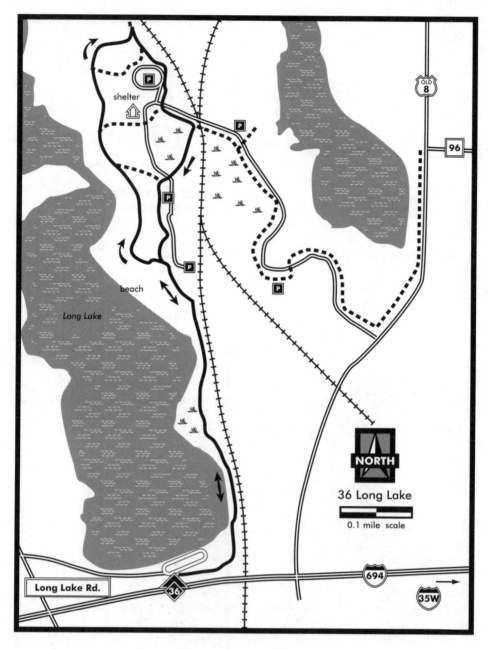

36 Long Lake

0.1 mile scale

lakeshore is wooded with tree branches arching over the water forming a continuous canopy along the shoreline. The right side of the trail is equally wooded but a railroad track and right-of-way has kept the undergrowth trimmed. The railroad track also marks the beginning of a signed interpretive trail tracing the history of the town of New Brighton (the park is located on the northern boundary of New Brighton). In its younger days, New Brighton was a thriving railroad town whose mainstay of commerce was the cattle industry.

Huge stockyards covering as large an area as the train yards themselves dominated the landscape along Long Lake at this time.

At Interpretive Sign 5 (on the left side of the trail) you see a description of the railroad turnaround and engine house that used to be on the site. A short spur trail toward the lake will reveal a few foundation remnants of these structures. Long since filled in, three large repair pits were also in this area. The engines would be driven over the tracked pits and repairs could be done underneath the train when needed.

Just down and across the trail another sign tells the story of the pump house that was erected to fill the huge steam engines with water. Just behind the pump house stood an 80-foot water tower which held 75,000 gallons for homes and industry in New Brighton. The foundation of that elevated water tower and pump house can still be seen just into the woods.

A bit farther, and again on the right, are remnants of three football-field sized ice houses that were used to store ice cut from the lake. A sleigh fitted with a large blade would score the lake ice, which was then cut and stored in the icehouse. Typically an ice house was insulated with sawdust, sometimes several feet thick. The blocks of ice were stored in layers with a layer of sawdust spread over and between each layer. This could keep ice well into the later months of summer. Over 8,000 boxcar loads of ice were cut, stored, and shipped from these ice houses each year.

The historic section ends just beyond the site of the ice houses where you'll see a very impressive scene: a majestic stand of cottonwoods. You literally have to crane your neck all the way back to see the tops of these towering broadleaf

trees. This is a very stately stand of fine specimens.

Soon after the cottonwoods and the historical tour, the trail comes out of the woods and into the developed area of the park. Groomed lawns, interconnecting paved paths, bath house, beach on the left—everything you'd expect in a well-developed city park. The trail blends into this urban setting but if you favor the left and keep heading toward the shore of the lake beyond the swimming beach, you will come to a paved path that does swing back along the lake for a short, but sweet, path through another wooded area.

This section is short-lived as it emerges into an open area. One other nature point along the way is at the first big intersection you pass while on this northern section. It's where the paved trail forks and a major route turns to the right. There is a triangular section of lawn where these trails meet that is guarded by a beautiful, spreading locust tree. As a former landscape-and-forestry graduate, this was another splendid specimen for me to enjoy.

Continue on along the trail paralleling the lake (almost impossible to see because of dense understory) to the spot where it comes out at the base of a big meadow knoll. The trail winds up to the top of the hill, past a large picnic pavilion next to the ball diamonds, and then intersects at a T. The left trail heads across a creek and out of the park to tie in to the Rice Creek West Regional Trail, which is frequented by bikers but open to hikers. If you feel ambitious, plan to take this out-and-back as far as your legs will carry you (the trail swings north and continues about 6 miles to the Elm Creek Park Reserve). For this hike, however, take the right at the T and head along the northern perimeter of the park, past the ball diamonds, and back to the center of the park. You'll come to several trails, all paved, that funnel into the main park area. Older maps show a trail to the left along another park road. That trail is right at curbside and doesn't allow you to come back into the park.

Taking the trail down to the beach area means you are again re-tracing your steps through the interpretive section in the woods as you cross through the beach area. It's a short section and it gives your mind a chance to conjure up images of the historic buildings you read about earlier.

Back through the 0.5-mile section of woods and you are back at the parking lot.

NEARBY ACTIVITIES

Interstate 694 is an effective link to other parks and hikes just minutes away by car.

#37
Mazomani Trail, Louisville Swamp/ Minnesota Valley

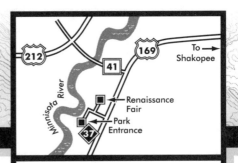

IN BRIEF

Enjoy this easygoing walk thorough a section of the nation's largest urban refuge, all the while passing through spectacular stands of hardwoods and swamp. The hike also winds through territory once inhabited by Wahapetonwan tribe and past the remnants of two frontier farmsteads.

DIRECTIONS

From Minneapolis, drive south on Interstate 35 West to Minnesota Highway 13 in Burnsville, then go west to the junction with US 169. Take US 169 south (right) to the intersection with 145th Street and turn right at the Renaissance Fair entrance. Louisville Swamp parking is about 100 yards beyond Fair entrance (drive past "Road Closed" sign when Fair is in progress in August and September). From St. Paul, take I-35 East to I-35 West in Burnsville, then proceed north to MN 13, then left (west) to the junction with US 169, and follow directions above.

DESCRIPTION

Before you start this loop, read the interpretive information on the kiosk at the trailhead at the end of the parking lot. There you will find a brief history of the first inhabitants of this area, the Wahapetonwan, a band of Dakotas whose name means "Dwellers." The trail this hike follows bears the name of their leader, Chief Mazomani. Known as "Little

KEY AT-A-GLANCE INFORMATION

Length: 4.5 miles

Configuration: Balloon

Difficulty: Easy to moderate; trail surface varies along gradual elevation changes

Scenery: Prairie vistas and large, mature swamp with islands of hardwoods; historic homestead buildings

Exposure: Half shaded from overstory; full sun in open prairies

Traffic: Trails shared with mountain bikers; less crowded in fall; some distant road noise at east end of trail network

Trail Surface: Varies from earthen to wide, mowed grass

Hiking Time: 2½ hours

Season: All seasons; wet in spring, particularly lowlands around swamp

Access: No fees

Maps: Available at information kiosk in parking lot or at refuge headquarters in Bloomington

Facilities: None

Special Comments: Textbook swamp in a prairie setting; homestead buildings and sites, coupled with historical information sets a mood reminiscent of *Little House on the Prairie*

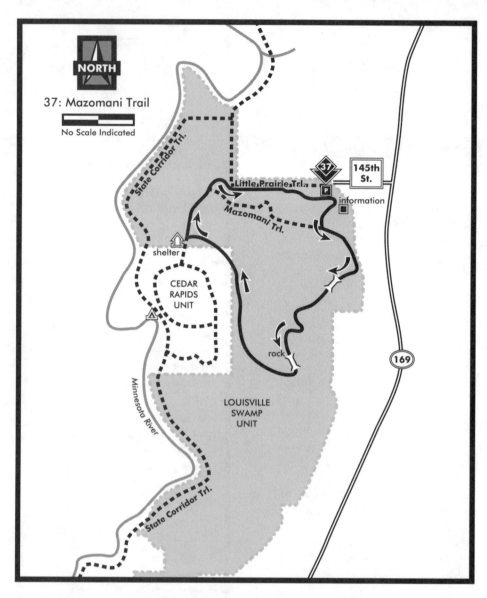

Rapids," their village was also the site of a trading post built by Jean Baptiste Faribault in 1802.

The Dakotas' native lifestyle in this primitive setting is set in contrast against two homestead sites along the trail: the Ehmiller Farmstead and the Jabs Farm. The main farmhouse of each family serves as a reminder of both the progress and the hardships these pioneers

endured hundreds of years after the "Dwellers" had first settled into the prairie/forested regions above the Minnesota River Valley.

Louisville Swamp is part of The Minnesota Valley National Wildlife Refuge—at over 17,000 acres it is one of the largest urban refuges in the country. The Refuge winds for over 30 miles along the shoreline of the Minnesota River

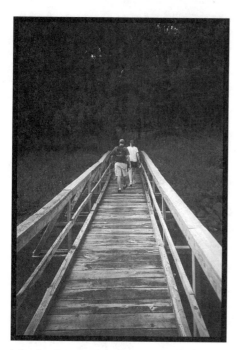

A footbridge along the Mazomani Trail through Louisville Swamp.

even more complete picture of homestead life on these prairies.

The Maz' Trail provides hikers the first view of Louisville Swamp by skirting above the edge of the prairie along a bluff. The trail then drops into the low floodplain-like area through which one of the drainages which feeds the swamp flows. An environmental note: draining swamplands for fields and other alterations have depleted Minnesota's marshlands severely in the past 150 years. A project at Louisville by Ducks Unlimited is helping to control flowage here to maintain habitat for wildlife.

During the spring or after heavy rains, expect this area to be quite muddy. A high overstory of mature silver maples and cottonwoods may keep this area muddy and wet long after a downpour. Expect an annoying number of bugs in the summer.

This is a multi-use park that allows small game hunting, archery, and groomed ski trails in the winter. Be respectful and watchful of these activities while you are hiking during those seasons.

Coming out of the lowlands, the prairie presents itself, at least in the fall when I visited, with a profusion of late season wildflowers and autumn colors. Especially profuse are the sumacs, thistles, and goldenrods. Islands of sumac, usually right along the trail, are common throughout the park, especially where prairie and woods transition into each other. The colors are bold and spectacular.

The trail continues southwest through across hilly terrain and representative stands of burr oak and white oak. The trail then borders a marshy area that offers the first good glimpse of the lake on the right. This is also the noisiest part of the park, especially in the fall when there are fewer leaves on the trees to buffer the sound of nearby highways.

This trail section is one of the more diverse in the park in that it takes hikers

before joining the mighty Mississippi. Numerous state, county, and regional trail systems interconnected along almost the entire length of the Valley. Collectively they form one of most extensive nature trail networks in the state.

From the parking lot, follow a short feeder trail that routes hikers to the trailheads of both the Little Prairie Loop and the longer Mazomani Trail. Take the route to the left: you can cut back along the Little Prairie Loop near the far end of the Maz' Trail if you want to hike this short loop back to the parking lot.

A short distance down the trail, you come to the Ehmiller Farmstead. Its main house, a two-story stone structure, is the most complete building still standing. Exploring the immediate grounds will reveal foundations and other remnants of structures. Later, about halfway around the loop, you'll see the Jabs Farm, a cluster of buildings that offer an

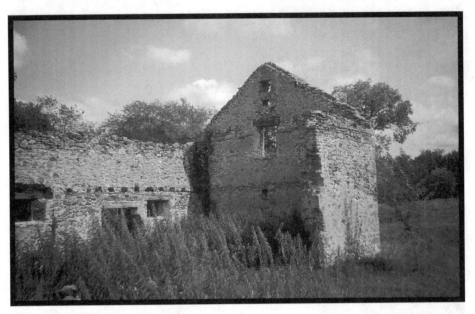

The remains of the Jabs Homestead.

through marsh areas, up along the highland meadows, and through mature stands of maples and cottonwoods along the creek.

About a quarter of the way along this trail you come to the first of two wooden footbridges in this wetter section of the park. The first bridge affords hikers good views up- and downstream. Keep on the watch for birds, particularly during spring and fall migrations. A list of over 250 species of birds that frequent the refuge is available where maps are obtained.

After a second footbridge, the trail turns into a broad roadway after coming out of the lowlands. It cuts through stands of characteristic hardwoods: oaks, birches, and sugar maples. As you come to the prairie again check out the huge boulder deposited by a glacier long ago. It offers the loftiest perch in the field and nimble climbers can get a good view of the surrounding prairie.

The trail follows the western edge of the swamp until it Ts with the trail junc-

tion at the Jabs Farm site. A trail to the left takes hikers onto the Carver Rapids Loop on Department of Natural Resources property. This trail loops around for 1.5 miles and features the Johnson Slough overlook. Another spur off of Carver Rapids Loop connects up with the State Corridor Trail that follows the south bank of the Minnesota River. About three and one half miles of the trail runs through the Louisville Swamp area.

Jabs Farm site contains a half dozen structures, from a complete stone barn to the standing walls of the granary and chicken coops. The Jabs family settled this area in 1905, working 35 milk cows on the 379-acre homestead. Plan to spend a half hour or so poking around the ruins and imagining life at the turn of the twentieth century.

The trail turns north at Jabs Farm and crosses the swamp across the spillway at this point. During the rainy season or after a prolonged rainy spell, it will be wise to check on the status of the spillway across Louisville Swamp. If its impassable, you will have to either backtrack the entire trail to this point, or use the Carver Rapids Trail and make a side loop hike of another four or more miles to get back to the Little Prairie Loop west of the parking lot.

Progressing over the spillway, open vistas in both directions present the swamp in all its glory. The gray ghosts of flooded trees and the expanses of marsh grass add character to the shoreline. Bitterns, herons, grebes, and a host of other waterfowl call Louisville Swamp home or use it for a resting site. This will be a good place to stop and observe birds and other wildlife for as long as time allows.

After crossing the spillway, the trail splits. The Mazomani Trail turns hard right and continues along the swamp, into the forest and back down into the swamp again. This section of the Maz is also the southern portion of the Little Prairie Loop. By staying to the left after crossing the spillway, you continue up along the western end of the Little Prairie Loop that takes you back to the spur trail to the parking lot. If you miss

this trail there is a second trail (a grassy roadway) that parallels the Little Prairie Loop back to the same trail intersection.

The middle trail (the upper loop of the Little Prairie Loop) will take you back through the upland hardwoods with a dense understory. Lucky hikers in the fall can enjoy wild plums growing along this trail. Be absolutely sure you know what they look like (little wild plums!) before you taste any. I like to bite into them and squeeze the pulp out. The skins can be mighty tart!

The upper trail of the Little Prairie Loop is about 0.75-mile long. It brings you right back to the parking lot just south of the information kiosk.

NEARBY ACTIVITIES
The entrance to Louisville Swamp is shared by the Renaissance Fair, held each August and September. Weekends will be crowded as cars line up to get into the Fair's parking lot. If you've never been, its a great experience. Also, the State Trail Corridor connects Louisville Swamp with other trailheads along the river.

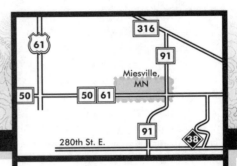

#38
Miesville Ravine Park

IN BRIEF

One of the enjoyable attractions at this park is the drive down into it. Its like a trip into Sleepy Hollow. Its a small park with two simple trails: one along the ravine and one along the river. Basic, yet unique.

DIRECTIONS

From the Twin Cities, drive south on US Highway 52 to Hampton. Go east on County Road 50 about 9 miles to CR 91 in Miesville. Turn right and go south on CR 91 for 1.7 miles to the intersection with 280th Street. Go left (east) on 280th Street 1.4 miles to the park entrance. Alternately: Go South on US 61 to CR 50, then go east to Miesville, following the above directions south from Miesville.

DESCRIPTION

As the county road leading into the park starts to drop down into the valley, you begin to sense that Miesville Ravine is going to be a bit rough, and totally quaint. This hike begins at the end of the north parking lot. There, a mowed, grassy corridor cuts through thick the brush understory and past tall cottonwoods lining the floor of the ravine. It follows Trout Brook for its entire length of just over 1.5 miles.

The first half-mile of the trail meanders through the large trees and gradually works its way towards the steep slopes

KEY AT-A-GLANCE INFORMATION

Length: 3.4 miles total (north trail is 1.6 miles; south trail 1.8 miles)

Configuration: The north trail is an out-and-back with two short loops, the south trail is a loop with two return options

Difficulty: Easy and mostly level, with a gradual elevation rise on the long loop on the south trail

Scenery: Mature stands of hardwoods and conifers, unobstructed views of Cannon River

Exposure: Mostly shaded on north trail; exposed to full sun on the south trail along the river

Traffic: Most activity occurs on the river, the north trail is less crowded

Trail Surface: grassy lanes, earthen hard pack with a few wooden walkways, can be muddy in sections

Hiking Time: 1½–2 hours

Season: All seasons

Access: No fees

Maps: Available at parking lot information board or www.co. dakota.mn.us/parks/ravine.htm

Special Comments: Not a park you happen upon, but worth the effort to find; this is the backcountry at its best—narrow roads, steep ravines, dense woods and a river

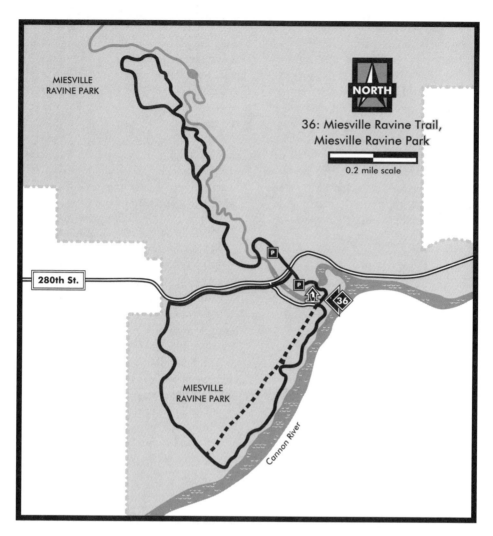

MIESVILLE
RAVINE PARK

NORTH

36: Miesville Ravine Trail,
Miesville Ravine Park

0.2 mile scale

280th St.

36

MIESVILLE
RAVINE PARK

Cannon River

of the ravine that line both sides of the small valley.

As you approach the stands of birch and maple, take the main trail, which splits off to the right before reconnection to the side trail after 0.17 mile. There is a wash-out from the creek that could be quite muddy during high water or after a good rain. This part of the trail winds through a dense growth of grasses, wildflowers, willows, and ash. The vegetation is very thick here, so it would be hard to get off the trail in this short section. This stretch of the trail should

explode with color in May thanks to all the wildflowers in bloom. Big willow trees and mature box elders provide the canopy overhead.

Continuing on, the trail joins back into the main path for another 80 yards to arrive at yet another intersection. This is the start of an enclosed 0.46-mile loop that encircles the marshy area up ahead. A wooden walkway assures dry passage over the trail at this point.

The park is home to beaver, raccoon, deer, wood ducks, ruffed grouse and wild turkey; so be on the watch. The trail turns back down the ravine halfway along the loop and continues on through more maples and ash. Signs of deer abound in this part of the park. As in the rest of this northern section, the pathway is level. That means you can expect soggy trails after rains.

In the area of the wooden footbridge, you will see green, segmented, tubular plants about two feet tall. These are horsetails, but are also called Indian scrub brush because their stems contain silica. A handful of the stems, when crushed, can be used as a scouring pad in camp.

Another plant worth mention, found in this and other parks, is the prickly ash tree. From a distance it appears to be nothing more than a sapling of common green ash. But upon closer inspection, you can see rose-like thorns all along its slender main trunk. It looks innocent until you pass too closely and feel its needle-like thorns.

Once you cross the footbridge, you are back on the main trail. It continues back along the route you came down, but stay to the right and you will pick up the 0.14-mile segment you passed earlier (when you took its 0.17-mile twin). The parking lot is about 0.4 miles further.

The southern half of the trail system continues on across the road to another parking lot. This leads over a bridge to a staging area for a local outfitter's canoe trips. The Cannon River forms the southern border of Miesville Ravine park and the first half mile of trail follows the river along its bank. During the summer, there will be steady but lazy river traffic in the form of canoes and kayaks.

This trail is a broad lane of mowed grass. Stately oaks, of the gnarly burr oak variety, stand like sentries between the path and the river. There are several areas where you have good, open vistas of the river and can make your way down to the river's edge.

At one of these you will see a rocky sandbar edging the channel. Immediately across from this area on the trail are wild plum trees. In September, their fruit is quite sweet and juicy.

After about half a mile, the trail makes a 90° turn back into the woods. Make another right turn and you can loop back to the parking lot on a straight, level trail. However, if you keep going straight past this intersection, away from the river, you can take the long way back: another third of a mile of hiking.

Go for it! This trail passes the remains of an old building and continues its way back up one of the ravines that cuts down to the river. As you climb up along the edge of the ravine, you'll pass through stands of birch and basswood. When you hit the dirt road, turn to the right (east) and enjoy the casual, 0.4 mile walk back down the country road to the parking lot.

NEARBY ACTIVITIES

Along the road and in the park, there is good bird-watching. Be on the lookout for gold finches, cedar waxwings, and indigo buntings. The staging area for canoes is a popular put-in spot for paddlers heading downstream a short distance to Welch Village.

#39
Minnehaha Falls and Creek

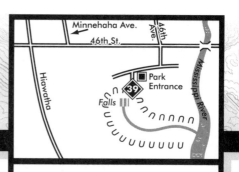

IN BRIEF

This is probably one of the most famous natural landmarks in Minneapolis. From the waterfall itself and the nearby statue of Hiawatha and Minnehaha, through the lush creek valley to the banks of the grand river of them all, this trail, as much as the numerous lakes, represents the City of Minneapolis.

DIRECTIONS

Much of this area is still under the construction (parking and entrances, for example). Access is available off of 46th Street/Minnehaha Parkway. From St. Paul, turn south immediately after crossing Ford Bridge. Watch for signs as entrances may change.

DESCRIPTION

I doubt there is a natural landmark in Minneapolis more popular than Minnehaha Falls. It's always at the top of the list for first time visitors. Prior to any hike along the creek below the falls, its well worth it to check out the falls from the upper walkways along the parking lot and across the bridge on the other side of the creek. You've got to see the statue of Minnehaha and Hiawatha—the love story that inspired Longfellow to write his famous poem, "Song of Hiawatha."

Once you've enjoyed the view from the upper falls area, you can descend one of the steep stairways that wind down either side of the creek into the basin

KEY AT-A-GLANCE INFORMATION

Length: 2.8 miles (walking up the Abandon Falls Glen easily adds another 0.25 mile)

Configuration: An out-and-back trail, with the option of a tight loop

Difficulty: Mostly level, but with some berms to climb

Scenery: Besides the falls, check out the golden walls of the ravine when sun bathes the valley rim

Exposure: Some shade up on top, fully shaded elsewhere

Traffic: The waterfall and easy trail attract bus loads in the summer; the trail spreads out the visitors, but the river bank brings them back together

Trail Surface: Road-like surface and hard pack; the alternate path through gets muddy when wet

Hiking Time: 1½–2 hours

Season: All season; access to lower area restricted in winter due to ice

Access: Newly designed parking lots require a small fee

Maps: Very hard to come by; copy the map in this book

Facilities: Concessions, rest room, picnic pavilion, drinking water

Special Comments: What's not to like about a waterfall? This is Minneapolis's most famous one!

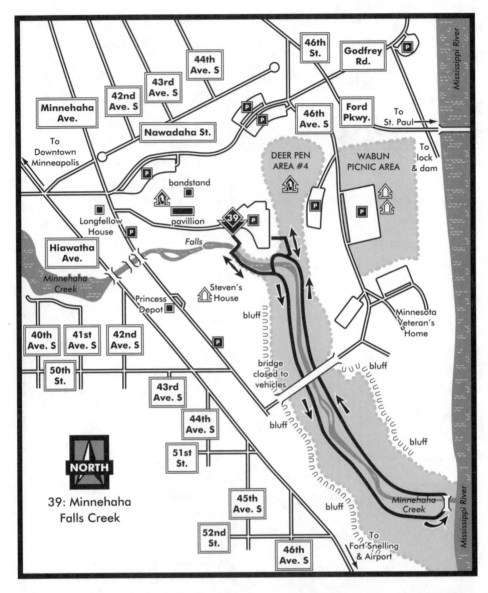

Map Labels:

46th St.

Godfrey Rd.

44th Ave. S

43rd Ave. S

42nd Ave. S

Minnehaha Ave.

Nawadaha St.

46th Ave. S

Ford Pkwy.

To St. Paul

To Downtown Minneapolis

DEER PEN AREA #4

WABUN PICNIC AREA

To lock & dam

bandstand

Longfellow House

pavillion

Falls

Hiawatha Ave.

Minnehaha Creek

Princess Depot

Steven's House

bluff

40th Ave. S

41st Ave. S

42nd Ave. S

50th St.

43rd Ave. S

bridge closed to vehicles

bluff

Minnesota Veteran's Home

bluff

bluff

44th Ave. S

51st St.

bluff

NORTH

39: Minnehaha Falls Creek

45th Ave. S

bluff

Minnehaha Creek

Mississippi River

52nd St.

46th Ave. S

To Fort Snelling & Airport

created by the falls. From various vantage points down below, it's much easier to see the mechanics involved in the formation of Minnehaha Falls. The harder limestone shelf over which Minnehaha Creek flows has worn back slowly over the eons. The softer sandstone below wore much faster and the water has created a gradually expanding bowl fifty feet below the limestone shelf.

Just past the pool created by the falls, a stone footbridge crosses the creek and offers great views back up at the falls and down through the stone embankment and tree-line corridor along which Minnehaha Creek continues on its last stretch before feeding into the Mississippi River about 1.5 miles south of here.

The path starts out as a wide walkway along the west bank of the creek. The

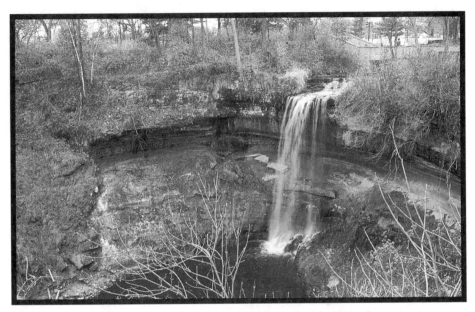
Minnehaha Falls has eroded the soft sandstone bowl beneath its limestone lip.

sandstone cliffs on the right have seen much wear and tear over the hundreds of years people have visited this area. Old timers may remember when a Native America in full costume would create sand paintings on one of the shelves of exposed sandstone. Today, graffiti, chiseled and gouged into the soft rock, provides a poor substitute.

The creek flows at a pretty good clip throughout the year— even in the dead of winter when the falls are frozen in a curtain of solid ice.

As the creek begins a curve to the right, another footbridge crosses the it again. Looking across the creek you'll see a long, sweeping, grassy glen to the north. This is Abandon Falls Glen. It's all that remains of an old channel through which the Mississippi River flowed before erosion along the main channel caused it to abandoned this course.

On your way down the creek's valley, you will be able to cross over and back two more times before reaching the river. At this point, the creek turns to the

right, away from the open field at Abandon Falls Glen. You can cross over and take the wider, more traveled path along the creek or stay on this side and walk along a non-maintained trail that gets muddy and cuts a tighter pathway through the trees. Both are very well defined and the creek serves as a common reference point.

If you are into wildflowers, stay to the right. In the springtime, this area is thriving with the yellow blossoms of marsh marigold and several other moisture-tolerant flowers. Because of some ground springs, this trail usually always has a few muddy spots, even in the heat of mid summer.

The creek travels a fairly straight course, only casually and occasionally meandering its way downstream. The trail parallels the creek, creating a pleasant promenade between the flowing water and the steep sides of the sandstone ravine. The trail is consistently flat for its entire route to the river. The south bank does have low and high spots and

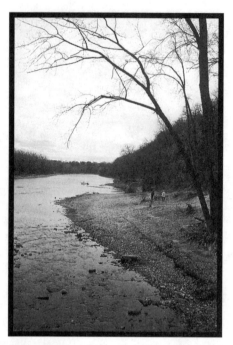

The confluence of Minnehaha Creek and the Mississippi.

derful frost patterns. As you stroll down the creek in the mugginess of summer, imagine the setting in the dead of winter and you will want to return.

The trail finally approaches the Mississippi, where the broad sandy embankment provides a wide view of the river through tall, stately cottonwoods. To the left are Lock and Dam Number One on the Mississippi River, the Ford Bridge, and Ford Motor Company's large St. Paul plant. To the south are the undeveloped banks of the Mighty Mississippi. In the summer, power boats cruise up and down this stretch continuously. You'll see where all those people carrying picnic baskets and fishing rods who you passed along the trail were heading.

The last footbridge on the creek right before it empties into the big river enables hikers to back-track along the opposite side of the creek they have just come down. Both sides of the creek are distinct enough to warrant a different trail route back to the falls. Each has points along the way where you can look up the face of the sandstone to see the unique erosion patterns in the formations. The golden sides of the sandstone cliff team up with a brilliantly hued blue summer Minnesota sky to form some incredible overhead views as well.

Minnehaha Falls is a peaceful corridor that acts like a special conduit between the activity of the city and the natural setting of the Mississippi River valley. No matter how busy it is up top, it's always tranquil at the water's edge.

NEARBY ACTIVITIES
Besides enjoying the amenities within Minnehaha Falls Park, check out the John Steven's house—considered to be the first house in Minneapolis. There is a flower garden, as well as more overlook opportunities, further along the upper west side, too.

requires better foot gear—and more cautious footing—than the main trail.

About half way down the trail, a few hundred yards beyond one of the stone footbridges and high overhead, are the towering and expansive steel arches of the Old Soldiers Home bridge. When you return back up top and if you have the time before you leave the park, walk out onto this structure and check out the views up and down the creek.

The trees and other plants along the creek are moderately lush, although its obvious that the tall, lanky trees strain to get as much sunlight as they can before those rays are obscured by the high walls of the ravine. Alders, dogwoods, cottonwoods, silver maples, and a variety of vegetation thrive in this deep ravine.

Walking down this trail in the winter is wonderland experience. The creek remains open in several spots, sending moisture into the air and creating won-

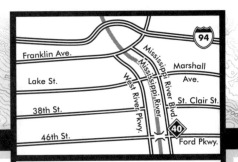

IN BRIEF

Hike along this pleasant urban trail that follows the bluffs along part of the definitive river system in North America. Pass one of the steepest and deepest sections of the Mississippi and visit one of the rarest native plant communities in Minnesota.

DIRECTIONS

To reach the Ford Bridge Access, take 46th Street east over the bridge, turn left (north) onto Mississippi River Boulevard. Parking is available two blocks north of the bridge. Other major intersections with segments of the trail are at Randolph, Summit, Marshall, and East Franklin Avenue in St. Paul. Main access points on the route in Minneapolis are at 44th, 36th, 35th, and Lake streets as well as Franklin Avenue. You can also enter the loop from Minnehaha Falls Park.

DESCRIPTION

Almost every park in this region is tied to the Mississippi River, either geologically, historically, or both. It's only fitting that one of the premiere hikes in the Twin Cities should be along this famous river corridor. The entire course of the Mighty Miss that runs through the Twin Cities is within the Mississippi National River and Recreation Area (MNRRA). The Mississippi Gorge section is one of my favorite sections because it's near the area where I grew up and it exemplifies all that this great river means to so many.

KEY AT-A-GLANCE INFORMATION

Length: 7 miles

Configuration: Loop

Difficulty: Very easy, flat except optional side trails

Scenery: Full vista of the Mississippi River along entire route with numerous incredible overlooks

Exposure: Western route shaded in morning, eastern route in afternoon

Traffic: Road traffic; high foot and bicycle traffic on entire course

Trail Surface: All paved along main course

Hiking Time: 2½–4 hours

Season: Open year round

Access: Plentiful parking at turnouts and along city streets, no fees

Maps: Available through the Mississippi National River and Recreation Area, 111 East Kellogg Boulevard, St. Paul, MN 55101-1256; possibly at the Mississippi Valley Wildlife Refuge Headquarters or at www.nps.gov/miss

Facilities: A few rest areas along trail, no other services

Special Comments: The Mississippi River defines Minneapolis as much as "10,000 Lakes" defines Minnesota; this is one of the best ways to enjoy the river

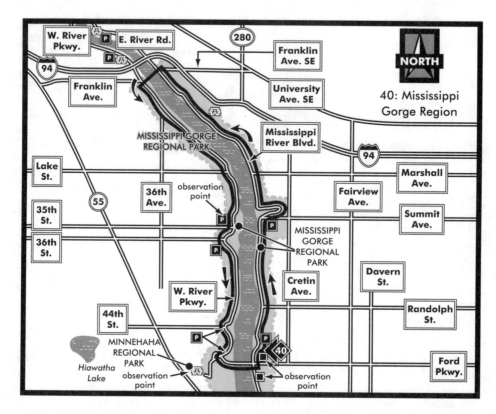

The MNRRA is also one of the few hiking trail networks that allows you to enter anywhere and exit at your leisure. There is ample parking all along the route and only your time and desire to stroll limits the amount of the 72 miles of foot trails/bikeways you can cover. This trail is well lit, too. Old fashioned street lamps line the promenade along the bluff, and the short stone wall on the river side of the trail adds to the quaint ambience of this stroll along the bluff. There are several places along the way where the trail opens onto a small glade, usually with yet another overlook to the river. The trail is consistent in its route—it's level and very easy.

The river presents itself beautifully all year long. Summer along any river is usually a relaxing adventure. With both sides of the Mississippi River open to hiking along the upper bank, you can hike in the shade of the western bank in the morning, and move to the shade on the eastern bank in the afternoon. If sun is what you desire, hike just the opposite.

Likewise, the seasons will affect the scenery along this hike. In summer, you'll find the trees in full leaf, and throughout fall the majestic oaks, basswood, and maples display a vibrant range of colors. Winter offers the most in the way of open vistas through the trees to the river below. You pick the season and the Mississippi is ready to provide the perfect backdrop.

For the benefit of description, this hike starts on the St. Paul side at the intersection of Mississippi River Boulevard and Woodlawn Avenue. As you walk north along the well-defined, eight-foot-wide sidewalk you are walking the very edge of the bluff, seeing the same river that settlers have seen for hundreds and thousands of years. From its source

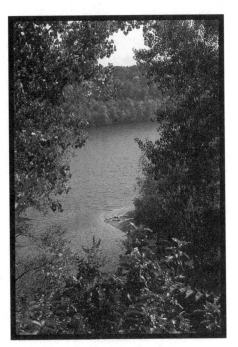

The bluffs along the trail offer majestic views of the river below.

at Lake Itasca to its outflow into the Gulf of Mexico, this is one of the steepest sections of the entire river valley. A few deep ravines have been cut perpendicular to its course and in some spots the road and trail follow them back from the river many hundred yards before turning back to the main valley.

Geologically speaking, this entire area was once a great inland sea. Only the tallest of bluffs were above water when the inland seas inundated this area. The Mississippi River cut a mighty channel through the bed of this sea to form the massive gorge it is today. Many of the other geological formations and characteristics of parks associated with the Mighty Miss have similar geological histories (Minnehaha, Hidden Falls, for example).

About a quarter of the way north along the eastern bank, the river makes a dogleg turn to the west. At Elsie Street, there is a small overlook that offers a

great photo opportunity, and a chance to capture the valley in all its early morning to mid-afternoon sunlit glory.

About ten blocks north of Summit Avenue begins the section of the hike designated as the Mississippi Gorge Regional Park. Across the river at this point is the western section of this park. If you are interested in the history of Minnesota's prairie wilderness, plan a visit to the Minneapolis side of the river.

Just past Summit Avenue a deep ravine cuts away from the river. This is typical of the type of larger drainages that once fed the river and helped carve these deep valleys into its bank. The trail continues on past Marshall Avenue in St. Paul, offering the option to take a shortcut and cross the Lake Street Bridge to the Minneapolis side and follow the river downstream. The trail continues north on the St. Paul side and soon passes through East River Flats Park. Farther on, past the Franklin Avenue bridge, you approach the University of Minnesota. Another entire section of this extensive trail, the Downtown Minneapolis section, begins here.

If you choose to cross the river at the Franklin Bridge, you can continue back down the Minneapolis side of the river to complete the River Gorge Loop. Your other option is to turn north and head to the downtown section along the West River Parkway, an extra 1.5 miles of walking.

Heading south back down along the river, the trail seems to meander more as it follows the bluff less closely. Here, too, are more opportunities to leave the shared pathway with bikes (as you do for the entire length on the St. Paul side) and venture into the bluff lands away from the paved trail.

These side trials are more adventurous in spots, but also a lot more demanding. Most are earthen trails, very slippery and muddy in the rains, some even impassable. One of these side trails runs nearly the entire length of Minneapolis section of this hike.

There is also the Winchell Trail and it begins right at Franklin Avenue and continues south to 44th Street. Most of the trail is paved and shared with bikers but many other sections are unpaved. One section cuts deep down to the shores of the river. This is the most primitive section of the trail since it descends the gorge leaving the developed part of the trail behind for a short distance.

One of the few remaining examples of a mesic (humid) oak savanna can still be found in the Minneapolis-St. Paul metropolitan area. Half of the remaining ten acres found in the city are located at the 36th Street segment of the trail. This is one of the rarest plant communities in Minnesota and is accessible via the Winchell Trail segment of the route.

A few blocks south, between 38th Street and 44th Street, the Winchell Trail runs parallel with the West River Parkway. There are trails off this main pedestrian-and-bicycle thoroughfare that enable hikers to drop down into the gorge section of the river.

Another ten blocks and you are back at the Ford Bridge and at a junction to take you to Minnehaha Park. You can link up with that hike (see Minnehaha Falls and Creek Trail, page 141) or continue back over the Ford Bridge to complete the loop. There's still more if you've the energy to continue south along the St. Paul side and hike the Confluence of the Rivers segment. See Nearby Activities below for more hiking options immediately south of the Ford Bridge.

NEARBY ACTIVITIES

Just south of the Ford Bridge is Lock and Dam Number One There is an observation area on the Minneapolis side.

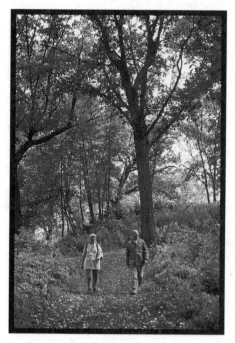

The forest is open and bright beneath towering hardwoods near the Mississippi.

Also, farther down Mississippi Boulevard, at Magoffin Avenue, is the entrance to Hidden Falls. It's a small falls with merely a trickle now, but once it probably had the roar of its brother across the river, Minnehaha Falls. Archaeologist have unearthed the remains of the giant beaver that once roamed the Mississippi River area eons ago near the falls.

A trail runs south along the river from this park towards the junction of the Mississippi and Minnesota rivers. This is the Hidden Falls-Crosby Farm Trail (see Crosby Farm Park, page 47). It runs along the river bank to the western boundary of Crosby Farm Park. There it joins up with the network of trails in the park and then continues on along the river to connect to the Downtown Saint Paul and West Side Segment of the great river recreation area.

#41
Murphy-Hanrehan
Park Reserve

IN BRIEF

One of the most rugged parks in the Hennepin Park system, this hike offers diverse terrain, challenging trails, and a great strenuous hike for hikers who want a good workout. This is a beautiful area with serious glacial moraine and one of the best stands of oaks in the Cities.

DIRECTIONS

The park is south of Savage and west of Burnsville. Take Interstate 35 East from St. Paul or I-35 West from Minneapolis to Burnsville. Exit on County Road 42. Go west 2 miles to Hanrehan Lake Boulevard (CR 74). Turn left and go west 2 miles to Murphy Lake Boulevard (CR 75). The entrance is on the left. The parking area and trailhead are on the left, just inside the park. The turn-out and gate for the alternate hike (Trail 12) is about 0.5 mile farther on left.

DESCRIPTION

Murphy-Hanrehan Park Reserve offers some of the most challenging terrain for hiking of all the parks in the region—but has the one of the shortest "hiking only" loops in the entire park system. The other network of trails is shared with cross-country skiers, horseback riders, and mountain bikers. To the park's credit, long-term plans do seem to indicate that some of the more demanding country within the park will be developed for multiple uses—and more hiking trails—

KEY AT-A-GLANCE INFORMATION

Length: 1.5 miles; alternate route is 4.5 miles

Configuration: Balloon; alternate trail is similar with options

Difficulty: Moderate to moderately difficult on steeper sections

Scenery: Very hilly with a solid stand of oaks

Exposure: Mostly shaded with some sun near the main trailhead

Traffic: Outside cross country skiing and mountain bike (i.e. spring) seasons, it could be very tranquil

Trail Surface: Packed earth, horse trails a bit soft, biking trails well worn, some exposed rocks and roots

Hiking Time: Main trail, 45 minutes; alternate trail 2–2½ hours

Season: Early spring for least amount of alternative trail use

Access: $5 daily vehicle permit, $27 Patrons Annual Hennepin Parks permit

Maps: Possibly at park and at www.hennepinparks.org

Facilities: Pit toilet, drinking water

Special Comments: The best trails must be shared with other users; birding should be good in spring, rich colors expected in fall

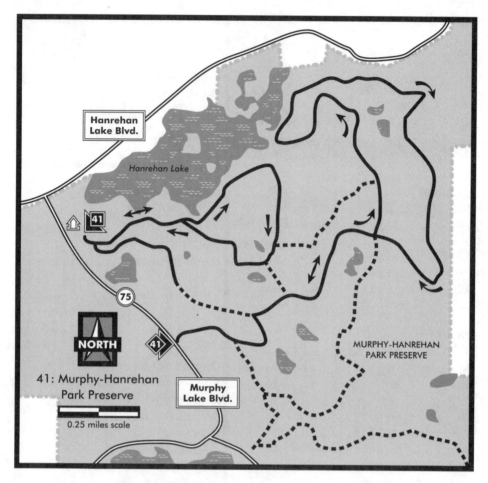

Hanrehan
Lake Blvd.

Hanrehan Lake

41

75

NORTH

41

41: Murphy-Hanrehan
Park Preserve

0.25 miles scale

Murphy
Lake Blvd.

MURPHY-HANREHAN
PARK PRESERVE

later. Let's hope so. With the exception of the mountain bike trail (the alternate hike described below), all of these trails can be used in the summer by bikers. During the summer, at least through July, the mountain bike trails are open for hiking. However, from August 1–November 1, these trails are reserved for mountain biking only. Bikers can get up some pretty good speed on the slopes, so hiking the wrong trail during the bike season could prove very hazardous.

What makes this park among the more topographically challenging are the steep glacial deposits—moraines—upon which this land developed. These moraines were formed during the fifth (and last) Wis-

consin glacial period. This created a landscape pock marked with sandy, conical shaped hills called "kames." Elevations in the park vary by over 100 feet. In addition to the hills, myriad lakes, ponds, and marshy areas have developed in the lowlands. The basins formed by the steep-sided kames are called "kettles."

From the parking area, hike east then take the left fork of the trail (Trail 1) and follow along the level ground south of Hanrehan Lake for about a third of a mile. It then forks again—stay left and start a climb toward the top of one of scores of kames in the park. The lowlands around the lake give way to some impressive stands of oak—one of the other natural features of this park besides remnants of the past ice age.

The predominant forest is of oak mixed with aspen. This growth is limited to the ridges and encircles some of the marshy areas. Open prairie-like meadows are more a southern park feature.

The trail simply loops back round for about a half mile to intersect with Trail 3 (posted). Take a right which will lead you back to the first fork from the parking area. You must retrace your steps for the last 0.4 mile back to the trailhead. That's it—the official length of the hiking only trails in this entire half of the park!

However, here is a great alternate route to consider: instead of taking the hiker-only trail, take mountain bike Trail 11 to the right. You can follow this trail east to the intersection with Trail 10. Trail 10 continues to the left and will connect with more mountain bike trails.

During your hike, be on the lookout for some rare glimpses of visiting songbirds and raptors. The park boasts an impressive bird list: loons, red-shouldered hawks, and two species of night herons. Other birds to look for are the rare Arcadian flycatcher, Bell's Vireo (another rarely seen bird), and scarlet tanagers. Also calling the park home are owls, mink woodpeckers, foxes, coyotes, and wild turkeys.

Trail 10 winds through stately stands of oak without a lot of understory. There are kettles in many places along the route as the trail winds around them or climbs to the top of one of the kames. This path continues for about 0.5 mile to intersection with Trail 9. If you are hiking in late fall, some of these trails will be closed so plan as you go.

At the intersection of Trail 9 take a left and start hiking on Trail 4. This is even more strenuous than before, but the corridors are wide and easy to walk. This trail cuts a serpentine swath through oaks growing high on the series of ridges formed above the northeast end of Hanrehan Lake. The trail does several severe cutbacks and forth before a long drop toward the lake. It continues around in a mile-long loop passing intersections with Trails 5, 6, 7, and 8 before connecting up with Trail 9 again.

In the summer you can continue on along one of the cross-country ski trails (if open). Both Trails 9 and 10 provide a longer loop that connects back to the corridor made by Trail 13, which in turn leads back to the road. Otherwise you will need to return along Trail 9, past the intersection with Trail 4 and head back out the way you came in. At the junction with Trail 11 you could continue on and come out at the park's headquarter area. This, in fact, is an option at the beginning of the "hiking only" trail, too.

I strongly advise hikers to carry a map. Without one you can take quite a few extra steps and turns before coming back to a familiar crossing. With a map, this tangle of turning trails coupled with hills and ponds can be one of the most rewarding hiking areas for shear challenge alone. You will find plenty of opportunities to test your leg muscles in this park.

NEARBY ACTIVITIES

You are within a mile of Cleary Lake. Modern and tame compared to Murphy-Hanrehan's ruggedness, it's close enough to be a great "after-hiking" area to picnic or casually walk down your muscles using the paved hiking pathway.

#42
Nerstrand Big Woods State Park (Big Woods Trail)

IN BRIEF

Big woods, incredible fall colors, a rich geological history represented by a waterfall—all offered on easy to moderate trails through stands of woods with ever-changing character. Its also the only place in the entire state to see the dwarf trout lily bloom in the spring!

DIRECTIONS

Head south on Interstate 35 to Minnesota Highway 19 east and go left into Northfield. Turn right (south) on MN 3, then left (east) on MN 246. Go right on County Road 40 to the park entrance.

DESCRIPTION

You have to know the human history of this park to fully appreciate these big woods. What remains is part of a pre-settlement hardwood forest that covered over 5,000 acres hundreds of years ago. When pioneers settled here in the mid 1800s they had the foresight to set up a small series of wooded lots that would remain unlogged. Theirs was a conservation effort based on utility—they wanted to make sure they had a sustainable supply of firewood as the woodlands fell to the clearing ax for farmland. These plots were marked out in what is now the center of Nerstrand Woods State Park. Created in the 1940s, this park preserved 1,280 acres of those wooded lots.

By happenstance I hiked this trail in the fall. It was a crisp, clear day and I had

KEY AT-A-GLANCE INFORMATION

Length: 3.1 miles

Configuration: Two stacked loops

Difficulty: Easy to moderate, however, fall leaf litter hides rocks and roots

Scenery: Stately trees—a mosaic of reds, maroons, and golden hues in the fall—and an open understory; small waterfall in a grotto setting along trail

Exposure: Mostly shade under the full canopy of the stately big trees

Traffic: Several places to get lost in this park; very peaceful

Trail Surface: Mostly grasses, earthen; uneven in many places

Hiking Time: 2–2½ hours average

Season: All seasons; good ski/snowshoe trails in winter

Access: Minnesota State Park fee system—$5 daily, $20 annual permit

Maps: Available at park headquarters or at www.dnr.state.mn.us/ parks_and_recreation/state_parks/ nerstrand_big_woods

Facilities: Visitor center with drinking water, rest rooms, showers during summer, campground with electric sites

Special Comments: Away from the freeways, surrounded by farm country; quite special woods

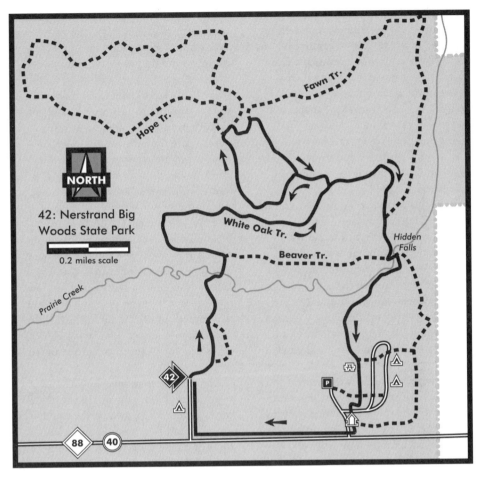

42: Nerstrand Big Woods State Park

0.2 miles scale

camped in the park, in the primitive group camp area. I left my tent behind and headed for the trail at end of the parking lot. The resulting hike heads into the northern section of the Big Woods, crossing Prairie Creek and connecting with network of hiking only trails.

You immediately sense the woodsy feel of the park by the mature stands of trees and lush undergrowth along the trail that leads down to the creek. At 0.4 mile the trail bottoms out at Prairie Creek. These are wooded lowlands typical of creek beds in the area. Oak Bridge crosses the creek here and hikers in the mood for a shorter hike can head to the right along the Beaver Trail for 0.4 mile

to Hidden Falls. But you don't want to cut the hike short, do you? The longer hike through more impressive stands and elevation changes moves back up the others side of the shallow creek valley along the White Oak Trail.

The trail climbs gradually back up to the ridge above the creek. The path is wide and easy walking. The woods rise up around you and a dense understory right to the edge of the trail guides you along under a spreading canopy of sugar maples, basswood, ironwood, elm, ash, and oak. The White Oak Trail connects to the Hope Trail turnoff at 0.4 mile from the Beaver Trail intersection.

This trail heads back west, like a switchback of the trail below, and enters into one of my favorite areas in the park. There is no understory beneath a dense stand of younger maples. It's a pathway between the golden maple leaves still clinging to the trees and those spread out as a thick, six-inch-deep carpet across the forest floor. It's a beautiful glen that sits in a shallow depression surrounded by the rest of the woodlands. It's one of many short segments of the trails in this park that has its own unique character. Equally impressive in the summer under a full sun, this section was likewise quite memorable in mid fall.

The Hope Trail section continues for 0.3 mile before intersecting with a short trail that cuts back into the woods. If you want to add an additional 1.2 miles to your hike, the Hope Trail continues on and climbs upwards to some grassy fields just west of the big woods. It eventually circles back down to connect to the far end of this same short segment.

Take the short cut, then turn right to follow the short 0.1-mile leg down to yet another junction. This time you have a choice of hanging to the left and following the upper sections of the Fawn Trail, a 1-mile loop that winds through the northeast corner of the park, finally emerging about 0.1 mile north of Hidden Falls. If you keep to the right and continue heading southeast, Fawn Trail continues down for 0.2 mile to a section of the Hope Trail loop taken earlier. It also leads on for another 0.1 mile to the White Oak Trail's eastern 0.3-mile leg before reaching a **T** intersection with the eastern end of the Beaver Trail. Take a left, cross the creek, and the falls are just ahead.

Prairie Creek reveals the heart of the forest floor at Hidden Falls. In geologic terms, the park sits on two nearly horizontal layers. The top layer is a 150-foot-thick layer of glacial drift. That layer sits on a layer of Platteville Limestone. Many of the river banks in this region have revealed outcroppings of this same limestone. The clay-like material visible throughout the park is this glacial drift. Hidden Falls is the only place in the park where the limestone is revealed— exposed by the cutting action of the creek through the drift. There are also sections along the bottom of the creek where the straw-yellow limestone is likewise uncovered.

The limestone has a much longer history. It was once the floor of a sea nearly 500 million years ago during the Ordovician period. During the last few ice ages much of this part of Minnesota was forever etched by the run-off from remnant melting ice. Prairie Creek's valley is a prime example of land sculpted in that era.

The area surrounding the falls is a series of exposed rock and low shelves of rock. It would be a great place to relax on a hot day. Because it is only about a third of a mile from the main campground, it is probably one of the most visited spots in the park.

The trail to the camp climbs a moderate grade through a thin stand of oak trees. This is along the eastern boundary to the park. The open meadow on the left may be what this entire area would have looked like had not the early settlers protected the big woods as they did.

The trail connects with the end of a campground loop and heads toward the entrance to the park. I choose this route so I could walk the last 0.4 mile along the country road that bisects the park. At Hidden Trail you could take the Beaver Trail back to the trail intersection with the trail from the group camp. It's the same distance, but the Beaver Trail follows the creek along its course above Hidden Falls.

Hiking this trail in the spring will reward hikers with a variety of wild-flowers including hepatica, Dutchman's breeches, blood root, young fern heads, and the dwarf trout lily (only found in this park!). There are lots of birds in this park, too, including blue-winged and Cerulean warblers, tufted titmouse, and blue-gray gnat catchers. Also make sure food and cooking items are secure in your camp. There are many bold raccoons in the campgrounds!

NEARBY ACTIVITIES

A working dairy farm, Big Woods Dairy is a special project run by a family that tends 50 dairy cattle on 80 acres using a rotational grazing system. Plans are to have the dairy farm open one day each year for visitors.

#43
Old Cedar Avenue Trail, Long Meadow Lake

IN BRIEF

An old bridge, once nearly covered by a modern "great flood" is the center point of a trail that is rather short, but offers exceptional bird viewing and provides access to several other trail heads. Its a great opportunity to enjoy the Minnesota River Valley's more open areas.

DIRECTIONS

The trailhead is at the base of a hill that dead-ends just before the bridge on old Cedar Avenue, south of Old Shakopee Road. Take the Old Shakopee exit off of Minnesota Highway 77 south of the Mall of America complex and head east (right turn at ramp). Turn left (south) onto Old Cedar Avenue and follow it down the hill as road curves left to the parking lot on the right.

DESCRIPTION

The Old Cedar Avenue Bridge hike is one of the most accessible hiking areas within the 34 mile stretch of wild parks managed as the Minnesota Valley National Wildlife Refuge. Its one of my all-time favorite places to go—especially to watch birds (and other marsh wildlife)—during the birds' spring and fall migrations.

There are three entrances to Long Meadow Lake's shoreline-tracing hiking trails. My choice is the Old Cedar Avenue entrance, which allows you make two out-and-back hikes from a central

KEY AT-A-GLANCE INFORMATION

Length: 3.25 miles

Configuration: Two connected out-and-back trails, with a 2-mile spur option

Difficulty: Level, easy former roadway of an auto bridge and avenue

Scenery: Mostly open expanses of the marshy Minnesota Valley

Exposure: Mostly full sun, some shade

Traffic: Popular spot for birders and joggers, but never seems crowded

Trail Surface: Old highway surface, wood-plank bridge, earthen path along the lake that gets muddy in rain

Hiking Time: 1 hour for out-and-back along bridge; bluff spur will add about 1½ hours

Season: All seasons, but not maintained in winter

Access: Parking ample; no fees

Maps: Large scale map of entire refuge available at refuge headquarters on I-494 and 34th Ave.

Facilities: None

Special Comments: I've been coming here for thirty years; I've always loved it, and usually see a new bird each time—there is something about the old bridge!

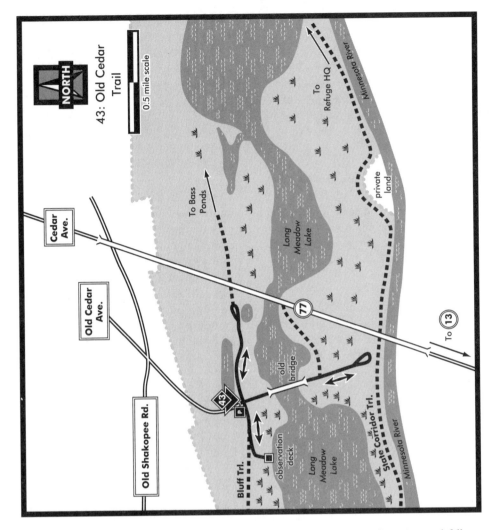

parking area. It's also the southern access point for the trail from the Bass Ponds (see Bass Pond Trail, page 16).

The parking lot at the Old Cedar Bridge offers three trail heads: the trail north to the Bass Ponds, the Bluff Trail that heads south for 2 miles to its terminus at Lyndale Avenue, and a short hike across the bridge to the Minnesota River, where even more trail options await the intrepid hiker.

It's so close and such a great viewing area, I suggest heading for the bridge as soon as you park your car. During the migration of birds each spring and fall, the old highway bridge at Cedar Avenue becomes a viewing platform for the northern reaches of Long Meadow Lake. The first several yards of the Cedar Avenue loop traverse the bridge. Step quietly onto the bridge platform, as you are walking over marshland habitat just a dozen feet below. It's sometimes possible to spot wildlife right beneath the bridge. Turtles will slide off logs, muskrats with slip under the water, and blue herons will take to flight, leaving you only a splash or a blur to ponder.

Egrets, herons, several species of puddle ducks, warblers, blackbird varieties, and elusive Sora rails are all common sightings along the bridge. A powerful pair of binoculars or a spotting scope with tripod will be a handy piece of gear for long stints observing wildlife down on the water or shoreline. Since the parking lot is only a few dozen yards from the bridge, it's a short walk with a hefty load of gear to get out onto the old iron trestle bridge with ease.

If you continue on across the bridge, you come upon a broad, street-width concrete lane, overgrown on the curbs with vines, bushes, and struggling saplings. Nature is slowly reclaiming this discarded ribbon of development. This corridor is another wonderful place to watch for birds. There are mature stands of floodplain trees (silver maple, cottonwoods) on the right between you and the marshy shoreline of Long Meadow Lake. On the left is an overgrown living fence of Chinese elm, small cottonwoods, willows, and other vegetation. Beyond this boundary is a grassy area, wet in the spring, but drier than the marshy area next to the lake.

A short distance down this lane is an unmarked but fairly worn path to the left. This cuts down into the upper marshy area, through a young forest of willow saplings to a point under the freeway bridge across the northern edge of the lake. From the base of one of the buttresses, this unofficial trail continues out to the shore of the lake.

If you choose to continue down along the overgrown roadway, you will come to another major intersection, offering numerous options. To connect up with the bike trails south of the river, go left up the bike/hike ramp and down the walkway built along the new Cedar Avenue (Minnesota Highway 77) Bridge across the river.

If instead, you turn left onto the trail that doesn't lead up the ramp, you will follow the Minnesota River beneath the bridge, eventually reaching the Wildlife Refuge Visitor Center (to protect nesting bald eagles, this trail is closed from February to July). The last option is to turn right and continue along the river about 2 miles. This unmarked path passes by the Black Dog power plant. It is totally undeveloped, primitive, narrow, and overgrown with vegetation, and the tall understory makes tight tunnel-like corridors at times. You'd almost expect to see river men in buckskin walking along this path, muskets and beaver traps in hand.

If none of these options hit your fancy the day you visit, retrace your steps instead, heading back to the parking lot to follow the next section of this hike, the Bluff Trail, which reaches Russell A. Sorensen Landing at its southern terminus.

At the west end of the parking lot the Bluff Trail enters a wooded area with a pond immediately on the right and a vista of the lake on the left. The trail continues back through the wooded shoreline, under canopies of towering cottonwoods down low and a some maples and oaks on the slopes that rise away from the trail on the right.

Several hundred yards into the wooded area, a trail spur to the left (there's a sign) heads out past the trees and out to the edge of the marsh-grass shoreline via a wooden walkway with an observation platform. Walk quietly and you will likely get glimpses of all the small sparrows and other shorebirds that live within these rushes. At the platform, you can look out over the lake and along both shorelines.

From this vantage point, you can only guess at what the rest of the refuge, extending for another 30 miles or more to the south must have to offer. Over 260 species of birds use this area each year, including nighthawks, wood thrushes, all the Minnesota varieties of vireos, and 75% of all the warblers known to reside or pass through Minnesota. Almost half the birds spotted in the refuge are believed to nest within its boundaries.

Geologically speaking this valley is the aftermath of a large glacial drainage known as the Glacial River Warren. It flowed from Glacial Lake Agassiz to form the Minnesota River Valley you see today from the platform. Many smaller streams were formed when the glaciers retreated. The Minnesota Valley is up to 5 miles wide and three hundred feet deep. Many of the streams that feed into the valley are spring-fed higher up in the bluffs. Like the other bluffs of the river valleys in eastern Minnesota, these are covered in oak savannas.

Return to the main trail and turn left, heading towards Russell A. Sorensen Landing. For the next 2 miles, the hike winds through the dense vegetation typical of low-lying floodplains along rivers. Giant cottonwoods and box elder tower over silver maple and ash. On the upper slopes of the bluff that edges the meadow, maples and oaks grow majestic. The trail winds up and over the modest but ever-changing roll of the land. Sometimes you start to ascend the slope only to be lead back down towards the marshes edge by the ever-winding trail.

Besides getting a taste of the ecosystem that typically borders a marsh, you are retracing history as well. Since the 1600's, fur traders plied the waters of the Minnesota River and hunted its banks for trade and food. During the two mile hike to the southern terminus, there are several places along the way to cut a path out to the edge of the lake for your own exploration.

Once you reach the other end, you can return along the same route or, again, have a shuttle car handy. The Black Dog Preserve, with its limited hiking, is just south of the bridge on the south shore of the river.

NEARBY ACTIVITIES

A hub for several trail options, the Old Cedar Bridge parking lot becomes the trailhead for at least three major trails along the Long Meadow Lake section of this great metropolitan refuge.

Cross the river and enjoy the Black Dog Preserve or catch the Bass Ponds trail to the north of the Old Cedar Avenue. Shuttling cars to end points on these otherwise point-to-point trails is a good way to cover a lot of ground without retracing your steps.

The Bluff Trail can be hiked from Russell A. Sorensen Landing, in reverse of the route mentioned above. Access this trailhead via I-35 West. Take the 106th Street exit, head east (right) to Lyndale Avenue, and turn south (right) to reach the Landing parking lot. The trailhead is at the end of the lot.

#44
Pine Point
Park Trail

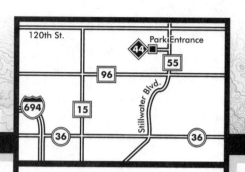

IN BRIEF

A small park with a robust hiking trail woven around the Willard Munger State Trail that serves as the backbone of this park. Pine Park is a major trailhead for the Munger Trail.

DIRECTIONS

From St. Paul drive north on Interstate 694 to Minnesota Highway 36 toward Stillwater. Take County Road 5 north through Stillwater to the intersection with SR 96. CR 5 becomes CR 55. Take CR 55 north about 3 miles to park entrance on left. Park at far end of parking lot near rest rooms.

DESCRIPTION

Pine Point Park sits close to the eastern end of the Willard Munger State Trail whose eastern terminus is only a few miles farther east of this park. While much of the park's trail use occurs on this wide, paved expressway for bikers, skaters, and hikers, it's the other network of walking trails that really introduces hikers to this park's character. Also, keep in mind that the trails at Pine Point, except for the paved trail, are shared with horseback riders.

This hike follows a very irregular, amoebic-shaped trail through Pine Point Park and captures virtually every area and amenity the park has to offer. Start right behind the information bulletin board to the right of the rest rooms at the end of

KEY AT-A-GLANCE INFORMATION

Length: 3.6 miles

Configuration: Three interconnected loops

Difficulty: Easy overall, with some hills, some soft and muddy sections; trails seem longer than on map

Scenery: Mostly upland forests with one big meadow and a few lakes short distance off trail

Exposure: Mixed full sun with dense shade

Traffic: Bicyclists on Munger Trail, hiking trails more secluded

Hiking Time: 2–3 hours

Trail Surface: Packed earth or mowed turf; wet in boggy areas

Season: All seasons, some trail segments part of cross-country network

Access: $4 daily vehicle permit or $20 annual regional park permit; reciprocity with Anoka and Carver County Park Passes

Maps: At bulletin board in park and www.co.washington.mn.us/parks/pkpinepo (*Note:* on website map CR 55 was mislabled as CR61)

Facilities: Rest rooms, drinking water, picnic tables

Special Comments: Some trails shared with horses; lots of biting insects in July

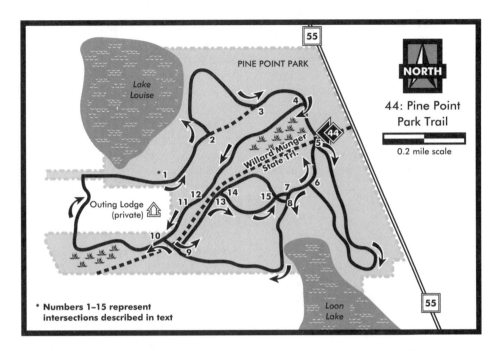

PINE POINT PARK

Lake Louise

55

NORTH

44: Pine Point Park Trail

0.2 mile scale

44

Willard Munger State Trl.

55

Outing Lodge (private)

Loon Lake

* Numbers 1–15 represent intersections described in text

the parking lot. The state trail leads right behind the bulletin board, but cross it and angle to the left. A few feet farther you'll see a six-foot-wide grassy pathway into the woods. Look for signpost (Intersection 5) marking the trailhead.

The trail is sandy and winds through oaks and spruce and a split stand of white pine on the right, red pine on the left. (A note of warning: I hiked this trail in early morning during mid summer and experienced hundreds of mosquitoes and deer flies!).

The trail bends to the left through a stand of red pines before swinging back around through a low area near the park's boundary. This lobe is about 0.3 mile out and another 0.3 back to the next intersection. At the end of the lobe the trail crosses a low-lying area that can be quite muddy after lots of rain. Birch, box elder, aspen, and spruce trees line the trail as you climb back up towards Intersection 6.

At Intersection 6 the trail intersects at a T, take the left trail towards intersec-

tion #7 on the map. You will come to Intersection 7 in about 50 yards down the trail. Keep to the left and go another 50 yards past intersection Intersection 8. You are now on a long, 0.4-mile lobe that brings you first along the top western edge of Loon Lake on your left and then swings around to skirt a large meadow on your right. There is a thick understory beneath a stand of aspen and oak between you and the lake so you won't see much of it from the trail.

This section of the trail is very narrow as it climbs up from the lake and out of the trees through a lighter stand of box elder and white maple. It has the character of a deer trail or worn hikers path in the north woods.

This trail intersects with the Munger Trail at Intersection 9. Take the paved trail to the left for about ten yards and then take a right into the woods across the trail to Intersection 10. If you imagine this entire route as a big, albeit irregular figure eight, you are now at the center of the 8, between the loops.

Follow the (muddy) trail to the left and pass a boggy area on the right. After a sharp right at a small pond (on your left), the trail now leads north and across a segment that actually lies outside the official park boundary.

You will come to a paved road that leads into the private Outing Lodge area to your right. Cross the road and continue on the trail cut into the thicket on the other side. There's no sign but it's very clear this is the trail. The trail continues as a narrow pathway through mixed buckthorns, box elders and red pine. The trees thin out a bit and as you pass a row of scotch pines (orange bark toward the top of a slightly gnarly upper trunk) you can barely see Lake Louise in the distance.

The trail comes out along the corner of the private property and then, according to the map, forks at Intersection 1. The right fork to Intersection 11 was impossible to locate on my hike, probably due to some light construction that may have obliterated the trail. It doesn't matter because this hike continues on along the left fork toward Intersection 2. As you approach Intersection 2, you'll see a field straight ahead. The trail to Intersection 3 loops to the north, first past Lake Louise, and then around the cropland before joining back up at Intersection 3. It's about a 0.3-mile loop if you go to the left, or about 0.15-mile if you cut straight ahead to Intersection 3.

From Intersection 3, the trail turns south and is only about 0.1 mile from the start at the parking lot. To gain extra miles and to see the interior of the park along the Munger Trail, turn right at Intersection 4 and head back into the thicker part of the woods. The trail cuts along the edge of a wet marshy area. Scores of frogs leaped across the trail here just in front of my feet.

This narrow "deer trail" continues through a tall stand of oaks. After the pond the trail literally sideswipes a gravel trail that parallels the Munger Trail. This gravel trail must be relatively new since it does not appear on the park map. Don't pay any attention to it as the narrow trail is more scenic and less crowded.

This trail meets the Munger at Intersection 12, but stay on the trail until you come to the signpost for Intersection 11. This trail, if taken to the right, takes you back to the corner of the private property at Intersection 1. Stay on your narrow path, past Intersection 11 and go another 0.1 mile to Intersection 10. You have just completed the upper loop of the figure eight and are back at the middle. From this point you technically backtrack along a trail that returns to the trailhead.

Take a left at Intersection 10 and cross the Munger Trail again, this time heading towards the meadow at Intersection 9. Turn left toward Intersection 13 about 0.2 mile farther. This segment follows along the southern side of the Munger Trail, passes Intersection 13 on the left, and continues on to Intersection 14, where it forks. Take either fork as they both end up at Intersection 15. From Intersection 15 you'll head to Intersection 7, which is a left turn if you've come from the left fork but straight ahead if you came up the right fork. Either way you want to go towards Intersection 7, where you will retrace a short, 100-yard segment of the trail you hiked much earlier (the section between Intersections 6 and 7). Now you are hiking it in reverse to head back to Intersection 6, where you take a left back up to the trailhead at Intersection 5, and the parking lot.

NEARBY ACTIVITIES

Stillwater to the south is full of shops. The quaint river village of Marine-On-St. Croix and William O'Brien State Park (see page 208) are a few minutes drive north.

#45
Red Cedar Trail, Wisconsin

IN BRIEF

Even though its a "state" trail/biking-and-hiking corridor, it's also one of only a few trails within 60 miles of the Twin Cities to the east and across the border into Wisconsin. Also, and more importantly, its course along the Red Cedar River makes it an especially enjoyable route to hike—replete with history, grand vistas of the river, and great scenery.

DIRECTIONS

From Twin Cities head east into Wisconsin on Interstate 94 and turn right (south) onto Wisconsin Highway 25 and drive to Menomonie. To reach the trailhead, turn right (west) onto WI 29 and go across the river, take your first left and park. To leave a shuttle car at the southern end, continue south on WI 25, through Downsville, to County Road Y. Take a left on CR Y and reach the parking lot on the right, just after crossing the bridge.

DESCRIPTION

Author's Note: This is the only "state" trail that is detailed in this book. While all state trail/regional corridors in Minnesota and Wisconsin offer many more miles of hiking and biking opportunities, those in the Twin Cities area either run along busier highways or cut through backyards or are part of former railroad right-of-ways. These are wonderful pathways in their own right. However, I think this one deserves

KEY AT-A-GLANCE INFORMATION

Length: 16.2 miles

Configuration: Out-and-back

Difficulty: Easy; flat with very few rises or dips

Scenery: Right along the river's edge

Exposure: Mostly full sun, some shade

Traffic: Bicyclists along the entire route, hikers vary by segment; popular trail during summer

Trail Surface: Entire path is hard-packed crushed rock

Hiking Time: 4H–6 hours

Season: All seasons; ski trail in winter

Access: No fee for hiking

Maps: Available at trailhead visitor center (old depot)

Facilities: Rest rooms, drinking water, picnic tables at visitor center

Special Comments: Watch for bicyclists; shuttling a car is a good idea; there are parking lots at each segment intersection

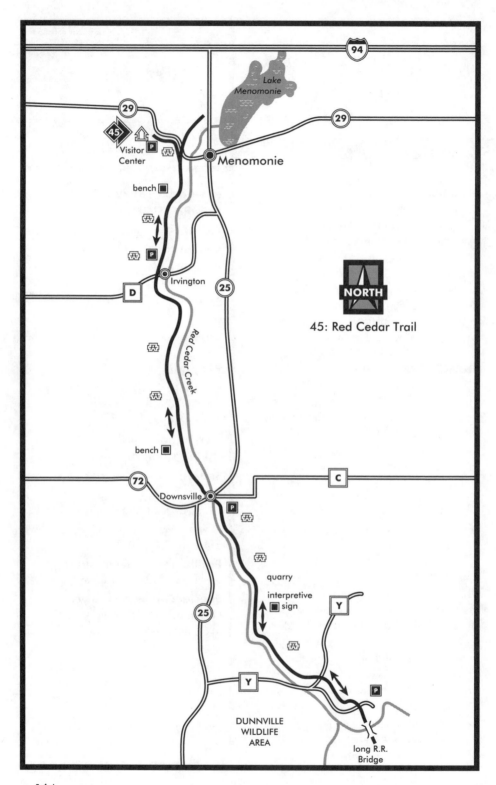

45: Red Cedar Trail

special mention because of its remoteness and beauty.

As most rails-to-trails paths, this trail was constructed on a railroad right-of-way; in particular, a section of the Red Cedar Junction Line which served the Knapp and Stout Company. At that time it was the largest lumber producing company in the world. Beginning in the 1870s, the line operated for nearly 100 years before being abandoned in 1973 when it was acquired by the Wisconsin Department of Natural Resources for trail development. The visitor center is the old railroad depot and fortunately this 14-mile course of the railroad followed right along the banks of the Red Cedar River.

This hike begins at the end of the small park adjacent to the Red Cedar Trail Visitor Center. A brief orientation of the trail's layout and history gives hikers an introductory perspective of the 14-mile trail. From the visitor center, head to the end of the parking lot, through Riverside Park on the visitor center grounds, and on to the trailhead. Each section of the trail is labeled according to the towns it connects along the river. The first section, 2.7 miles, runs from Menomonie to Irvington.

This is river country, the woods along the river's edge are typically silver maple, box elder, and their representative understories of sumac and hazelnut and myriad other vegetation. Higher points along the river encourage oaks and other, harder sugar and red maples to take hold.

After roughly 1.1 miles, you'll come to a large rock face on the right, rippling with a constant oozing of water along its entire face. In the summer these "weeping rocks" promote a healthy covering of ferns that cling to the walls. The area is actually called the Ice Palisades because in the winter, this water freezes forming

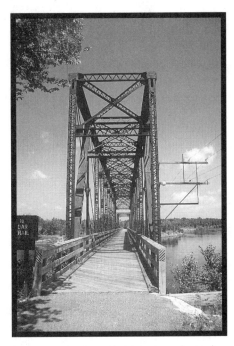

A converted railroad bridge along the Red Cedar Trail.

a wintry shroud of ice over the entire cliff face.

Geologically speaking the Red Cedar River is in that area of Wisconsin known as the Driftless Area. That's the area where the most recent glaciers from the last Ice Age failed to cover the land. It's terrain is therefore more rolling and otherwise different from the scoured and scored landscapes to the north.

Some maps talk of a Devil's Punch Bowl formation a bit farther down from the Palisades—on the right side just before coming into Irvington. I could not find the site. Perhaps poking more thoroughly through the thick undergrowth along this section would reveal it to bushwhackers.

The next section is 4.3 miles long and continues toward Downsville. The countryside changes a little bit along this section as it opens up more into farm country and marshes. About 1.5 miles down this section is Varrey Creek. Archaeological digs have uncovered 3,000-year-old arrowheads in this area. Ironically, the name "Red Cedar" isn't native in origin at all. It's name comes from finding one red cedar tree floating in the river during the time French traders were exploring this area.

At Downsville the trail crosses the river and heads down its eastern bank. This section is called the Dunnville section and adds another 4.2 miles to the trail's length. The trail isn't as close to the river as it has been. This section is noted for the number of quarry sites found about half way down this section. An interpretive site at Mile 10 marks the site of the Dunnville Sandstone Quarry.

A mile farther and you'll come to a bend in the river and a picnic site. There used to be petroglyphs near this site but they have long since been destroyed. They still may appear in some references and on some maps.

At Dunnville you cross County Road Y and enter the Dunnville National Wildlife Refuge. A parking lot across the bridge (take a right at CR Y) can serve as the southern terminus of this trail since it's a good place to park a car if

you are making this a one-way hike with a car shuttle. The trail does continue on for another 2.5 miles to a long railroad bridge over the river. Just upstream from this bridge is the confluence of the Red Cedar with the Chippewa River, a moderate tributary to the Mississippi River from Wisconsin.

It's worth the walk to see this old, narrow bridge that looms across the river. There is also an expansive sandy beach down the trail to the right, accessible just before you approach the bridge, that is a popular resting place for hikers and bikers. You'll even see waders and swimmers cooling off at this wide, gentle bend in the river.

From the railroad bridge the trail continues another 26 miles as the Chippewa River State Trail. The Red Cedar portion ends and you must backtrack to either the parking lot at CR Y, or all the way back to Menomonie. There is also designated parking at Irvington for dropping a car at that point along the trail.

NEARBY ACTIVITIES
Check your road map—on the way back to Minnesota you have a few options to enjoy other trails in Wisconsin's parks.

#46
Rice Creek Chain of Lakes Regional Park Reserve

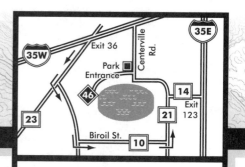

IN BRIEF

A chain of seven lakes with broad, paved trails nicely wrapped around each provides hikers of every age—and even those confined to wheelchairs—a great opportunity to experience a sampling of Minnesota's natural resources.

DIRECTIONS

From north of St. Paul and from Minneapoli, take Interstate 35 West towards Centerville. Turn right (south) at Exit 36. Drive approximately 1 mile to Aqua Lane, turn left (east) to the first parking lot near the lake. Trail just north of lot. From St. Paul, take I-35 East north to Exit 123 (C.S.A.H. 14). Turn left (west) and follow past Centerville Road (C.S.A.H. 21) to campground/ park's east entrance. Turn left and follow main park road to its end. Park in lot near boat launch. Trailhead is just across the road, opposite the lot.

DESCRIPTION

If a nicely groomed, modern developed park setting is to your liking, you'll love the setting at Rice Creek. This is about as new as parks get, some of the trails are not even laid out yet. However, if you want a taste of northern Minnesota over the course of a very casual, extremely easy 2-mile walk, this is the park for you.

Currently there are only a few "official" trails for hiking in this park. Many more have been designated and will be

KEY AT-A-GLANCE INFORMATION

Length: 2 miles

Configuration: Out-and-back

Difficulty: Easy throughout, on level, bituminous walkway; some primitive trails are narrow, with roots exposed

Scenery: Marshes and lowland forests connect the lakes, a real "northern" Minnesota setting

Exposure: Main trail is open with no canopy for shade, primitive trails through wooded areas

Solitude: A people's park that invites bike riding, hiking—expect to see families

Trail Surface: Paved; better than some streets in the Twin Cities

Hiking Time: 45–60 minutes

Season: All season; flat terrain for skiing/snowshoeing in winter

Access: $4 daily use fee, $20 annual permit; reciprocity with Carver and Washington County Park Passes

Maps: Available at gate

Special Comments: This park is till under development and overflowing with "newness"; many additional trails are yet to be marked or paved

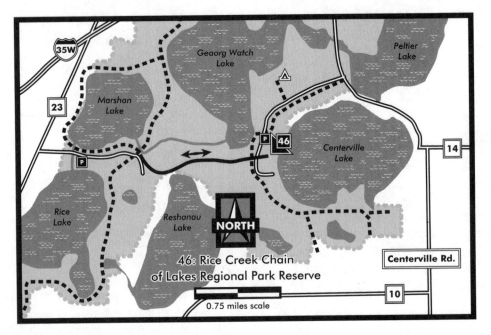

46: Rice Creek Chain
of Lakes Regional Park Reserve

0.75 miles scale

developed as part of the park's Master Plan. There already is a bike trail along the main road and connecting developed areas, but this is along the open stretches of the park that you can just as easily drive down. To get out and see the park on the paved hiking trail that cuts through the center of this park, you need to begin at the Centerville Lake parking lot. (Since this is a pretty easy out-and-back trail, just reverse directions if you parked off of Aqua Lane.)

This trail begins at an intersection of the main bike trail, across from the parking lot. This eight foot wide, bituminous bike path/hiking trail showcases what to expect from trails yet to be opened as it bisects the park and lake chain right in the center. If you have a friend or family member confined to a wheelchair, this is one of the easiest parks for them to enjoy, because it's trails are level and designed with very gradual curves.

There are no surprises on this otherwise pleasant path. A ten-yard swath of grass found on either side of the path

adds additional width to this already wide corridor as it cuts through tall, narrow aspens mixed with ash and willows. It's like being in a neighborhood park. In fact, this trail cuts into the golf course and gives you the option to continue on or return. Instead of continuing, make this a short one.

Don't let the groomed and trimmed feel of the park fool you. There is a "wilder" side to the park in the natural areas that border this route all the way to the golf course (OK, the "wildness" is short-lived!). Most of the lower areas are marshland with a profusion of cattails and alders lining their edges.

Along this very defined path are rough trails etched into the ground that disappear into the understory, particularly where there are natural routes around the many lakes. Eventually you will be able to loop around almost all the lakes and connect back to the main road or continue on to interconnected corridors that will make up the Rice Creek Regional Trail system. In all, three junctions of the regional system will be accessible from this park.

This is a casual birder's park. Most of the views of marshes through the trees will reward visitors with sightings of egrets and great blue herons as well as the ubiquitous flocks of mallards and other common puddle ducks.

I found another interesting trail in this park, one designated but not yet developed or officially marked. Upon returning to the main park road, and before crossing the street back to the parking lot, turn rightand go about a half block. This trail follows the edge of the meadow lands between Centerville and Reshanau Lakes It laces in and out of the trees and offers a glimpse of trails to come.

Dogwoods, willows, alders, and understory plants that like more moisture and more shade abound in the wooded sections between the lakes. I noticed scores of very active goldfinches during a visit to this park in August. During the spring and fall bird migrations, I suspect this is a great stop-over resting place for scores of other species, too. While in its undeveloped stages, these random trails are all perhaps fair game and due to be upgraded to full status as official hiking trails. Feel free to explore.

There is enough going in this park, now and in the future, to make it a very popular recreation area. Besides the golf course and the developing trail network, there is also a five-lake canoe route that runs from the collection of lakes at the southwestern end of the park. The canoe route is about 8 miles long with two short portages.

This is the hike to take when you're in the area and don't have much time but don't want to miss the sights and sounds reminiscent of more secluded, less developed hiking areas.

NEARBY ACTIVITIES

Golf and canoeing. Once trails develop, there should be many nice loops, balloons and out-and-backs upon which to hike.

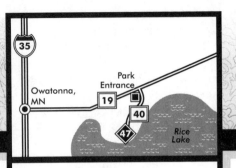

#47
Rice Lake State Park

IN BRIEF

Whether you are a bird watcher, pioneer historian, or interested in ice age geology, you'll find that Rice Lake has much to offer. Rice Lake has one of the most complete and richest histories of all the parks in this area—and in the entire state park system. Hike this park during the early spring bird migrations for an added treat!

DIRECTIONS

Head south from the Twin Cities on Interstate 35 to Owatonna to Exit 42, (County Road 19) Continue east (left) about 14 miles on CR 19 to park entrance. Turn left into park, then take second right to boat ramp area.

DESCRIPTION

This loop connects most of the areas in the park, so you could start just about anywhere. For our purposes, this hike begins at the canoe ramp. Should you want to take a relaxing paddle around the lake after the hike, bring your own boat or rent one there.

From the boat ramp, head south, observing along the way the young oaks and maple woodlands extending back from the marshy shorelines around Rice Lake. The marshy outline of the lake extends around the southeast edge of the park's developed area (shelter, picnic grounds, playgrounds). The trail hugs the shoreline and continues through more

KEY AT-A-GLANCE INFORMATION

Length: 2.2 miles

Configuration: Loop with options

Difficulty: Easy; fairly level around lake shore, modest elevation changes elsewhere

Scenery: Pleasant woodlands with lake in background

Exposure: Mostly full sun, some shade

Traffic: Late fall is very quite, expect more activity in summer; it's a small park

Trail Surface: Packed earth, some paved walkways on "shortcuts"

Hiking Time: 1–1¼ hours

Season: All seasons; spring for birds, fall for colors, winter for skiing

Access: $4 daily vehicle permit, $20 annual state park permit, or $12 annual permit for disabled persons

Maps: Available at park headquarters or at www.dnr.state.mn.us/ parks_and_recreation/state_parks/ rice_lake

Facilities: Pit toilets available at several places along the hike, rest rooms at campground, water available at 0.3 and 1.3 miles into the hike

Special Comments: Trail starts at boat launch, bring your canoe

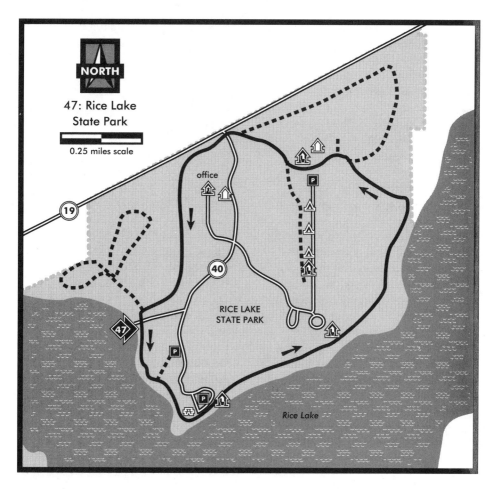

47: Rice Lake
State Park

0.25 miles scale

office

RICE LAKE
STATE PARK

Rice Lake

mature oaks and maples. It's a three-foot-wide, level earthen trail that gets as close to the water's edge as possible. It's about 0.3 of a mile from the boat launch to the picnic area and another 0.3 mile to the next trail junction which cuts back up to the drive-in campsites. It also connects with one of the trails leading to the walk-in camps located just off a park road in the center of the park. Stay along the lake for this longer hike.

If you are visiting during Minnesota's spring bird migration season, you may want to spend some time in this park, either at the camo bird observation platform at the picnic/playground area or nestled down along the shoreline some-where. Rice Lake is one of the largest bodies of water between this part of the state and the Mississippi River. Be on the lookout for whistling swans, Canada geese, snow geese, blue geese, a variety of diving ducks, pied-billed and Western grebes. Also, Black terns nest in the park. Seven species of woodpeckers have been spotted in the park—including the large pileated woodpecker.

This is a shallow lake, formed out of shallow drift left by the Kansas Ice Age which was one of four advances of ice across Minnesota. Rice is also one of the headwaters of the Zumbro River. Its outlet forms the South Branch of the Middle Fork.

Also of note is the bedrock in this area, formed over 500 million years ago when a shallow sea covered most of North America. The sediment deposited was hundreds of feet thick. That deposit hardened and is the same material found in the bluff lands to the east—further cut by the Mississippi River.

The trail continues to cut through oaks and maples as it follows the lake up into the higher meadows. The trail ascends gradually from its low course along the edge of the lake. Rice Lake sits in an area of incredibly rich soil, so rich that many of the oak-barren meadows were converted to agriculture. The meadows the trail meanders through now are only reminders of the type of country that used to exist here. The true reminders are the burr oaks, the dominant species of oak barrens that once stretched from Rice Lake down into Iowa.

From the junctions with the camping area the trail continues for another 0.6 mile to another junction in the meadows which offers an option—a 0.7-mile loop that winds around the northern section of the park's east side before linking back around on itself just before the road. If you stay to the left of this junction, you'll hike another 0.2 mile to the northern intersection of a trail that cuts back to the walk-in camps.

As the trail crosses the main park road you can choose to follow it back or continue through more meadow country. Either way is about 0.6 mile and ends back at the boat ramp. If you take the trail, you can access an additional 0.8 mile of trail, located just before you reach the ramp. These two loop trails circle through some swampy areas (the shorter loop) or back out onto the meadows (a 0.4-mile loop). These and a few other main trail segments are ski trails in winter.

Nearby Activities
The park literature describes the local history, including an old town site, stagecoach line, and other interesting pieces from the past preserved in the nearby towns and neighborhoods.

#48
Rum River Central

IN BRIEF

One of several hiking opportunities along the popular Rum River, this hike follows a major bend in the river and offers a short but scenic hike through central Minnesota river lowlands.

DIRECTIONS

From Minneapolis, take US Highway 169 north to Anoka. In Anoka take County Road 47 (right) north about 6 miles to 179th Lane NW. Turn right and drive for about a mile to CR 7. The park entrance is right across the street. Take the park road to the Visitor Contact Station, then follow the road past the horse-trailer parking lot to the next parking lot on the left, about 0.3 mile into the park.

DESCRIPTION

This is primarily a horseback riding park but the trails are designated for horses and hikers. There is a separate bike trail, too. Both parallel the river. Start from the north end of the parking lot and head to the left. This area has marshy lowlands but soon the trail rises into stands of hardwoods and winds through oaks, basswoods, birch, and even some evergreens. Songbirds seem to be particularly active and vocal in this section, too.

The trail passes through some open areas as it crosses the road near the entrance to the park. From there the trail

KEY AT-A-GLANCE INFORMATION

Length: 3 miles

Configuration: Loop

Difficulty: Easy; level walking but trail sometimes soft and muddy

Scenery: Many views of the river, lowlands, and some meadows with wildflowers

Exposure: Shady along the river, sunny in the uplands of meadows

Traffic: Expect weekends to be most active

Trail Surface: Earthen, some well churned by horses

Hiking Time: 1½–2 hours

Season: Some trail sections reserved for skiers in winter

Access: $4 daily vehicle permit or $20 annual county park permit; reciprocity with Washington and Carver County Park Passes

Maps: Available at the park or at www.anokacountyparks.com/qlinks/parks

Facilities: Picnic area with pavilion, rest room, drinking water, playground

Special Comments: Best to choose this park during drier seasons

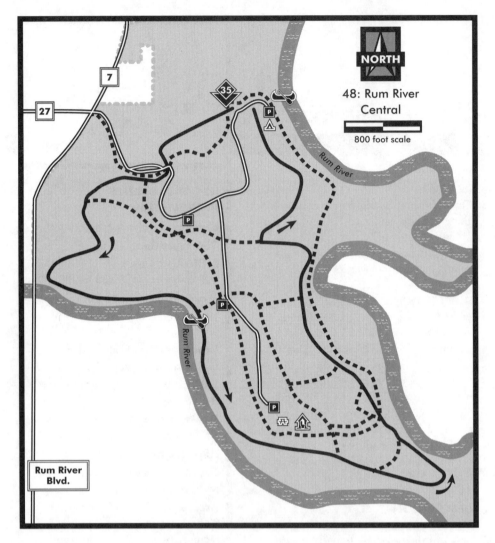

48: Rum River Central

800 foot scale

Rum River

Rum River

Rum River Blvd.

meanders through oak savanna areas and more trees and marshy areas on its way to the river. About a half mile from the entrance to the park, you will meet up with Rum River and be able to walk along it for nearly a mile.

The Rum River flows out of Mille Lacs Lake about 60 road miles to the north. The Rum winds over an additional 40 miles after leaving the park on its way to the Mississippi River. The river forms the southern, eastern, and northern boundaries of this park as it

meanders for about 4 miles through this area.

Once walking beside the river bank, you will soon come to the walk-in canoe launch area. For the next 0.8 mile or so, the trail meanders along a peninsula-like strip of land, passing through a variety of vegetation common to floodplains as well as some of the higher growth from those wet areas.

The river nearly doubles back on itself at this point along the southern boundary. The banks are lined with box elder

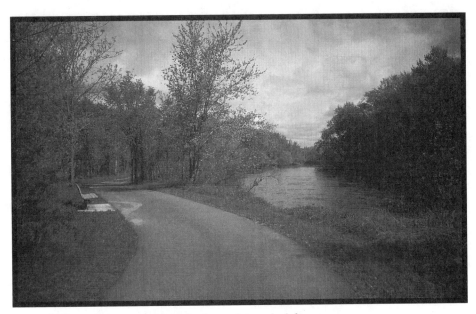

The level bike trail along Rum River; the footpath is to the left.

and ash trees with a few cottonwoods common to Minnesota's river country.

Following the lead of the river, the trail turns abruptly back along a hairpin turn that heads north. About 120 yards after the trail loops back, you will cross the paved bicycle path. At this point the two trails (bike and horse/hike) parallel each other as they follow the east bank of the river upstream. The bike trail and horse path are separated by a thin corridor of brush and thickets, but there are several places hikers could poke through to get glimpses of the river.

Soon after crossing the bike trail, there is another horse trail to the left. Stay on a straight course and continue to follow the river. About 0.2 mile farther, you'll come to another horse trail on the left. Again opt for the trail straight ahead.

The trail rises about 30 to 40 feet as it starts to turn away from the river. At this point you will notice that the oaks and basswoods are quite a bit bigger. The forest is more like upland hardwoods. The

basswood is a dominant species here. It's the tree with the big heart-shaped leaves. It's also called linden when used for landscaping.

You will soon come to an intersection. This is another junction with the paved bike trail. The hiking trail continues across the paved trail for about 500 feet before taking a sharp turn away from the river and into the heart of the park. The trees are bigger here, denser canopies comprised of large box elders.

Another 500 feet beyond this last intersection, the trail curves sharply to the right and heads back toward the Horse Trailer Parking lot. However, as a hiker, you should turn right about 0.1 mile down this stretch. This will lead you past the canoe campsite and back to the parking lot and trailhead.

NEARBY ACTIVITIES
Visit Rum River North, which is just up the road, and Elm Creek Reserve a few minutes south for more hiking

possibilities. The town of Anoka offers restaurants and other local, small town shopping. Also consider canoeing along the Rum River, a great half day paddle is possible from the Rum River North Park by St. Francis, down to this park. There are no canoe rentals or shuttles available so you'll have to have your own gear and means of getting back to your car.

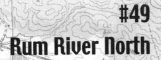

#49
Rum River North

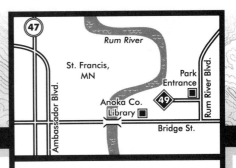

IN BRIEF

One of three county parks along the Rum River, this northern extension lies on the east bank of the river, providing excellent views of the water while passing under a thick canopy of northern hardwoods.

DIRECTIONS

From Minneapolis, drive north on US Highway 169 to Anoka. Take County Road 47 north (right) to St. Francis. In St. Francis, turn right onto Bridge Street off of Ambassador Boulevard and take the bridge over the Rum River. Take next left after Anoka County Library (on left) onto Rum River Boulevard. Go 500 feet and take left into park. Turn right after 200 feet and park in lot next to main pavilion.

DESCRIPTION

The Rum River is one of those rivers with a northerly feel to it that is close enough to enjoy with only a short drive from the Twin Cities. I spent many a weekends along its banks as a Boy Scout.

The trail starts at the main pavilion next to the parking lot. Basically the trail follows the river as it forms the boundary for the western edge of this park. Both ends of the trail loop back onto the mail trail to provide about 2 miles of hiking within the park's boundaries.

From the pavilion, hike north along the paved trail that joins the river at a T

KEY AT-A-GLANCE INFORMATION

Length: 4.4 miles

Configuration: An elongated figure eight

Difficulty: Very easy; few changes in elevation, smooth trail surface

Scenery: Trail follows river for most of route through modest overstory of trees

Traffic: Promoted as a multi-use park, lots of activities all year long

Trail Surface: 1-mile loop is paved; wooded section along arm is packed turf

Hiking Time: 1½–2 hours

Season: All seasons, could be very pretty in winter

Access: $4 daily vehicle permit, $20 annual regional park permit; reciprocity with Washington and Carver County Park Passes

Maps: Available at the park or at www.anokacountyparks.com/qlinks/parks

Special Comments: Access to park is right in St. Francis

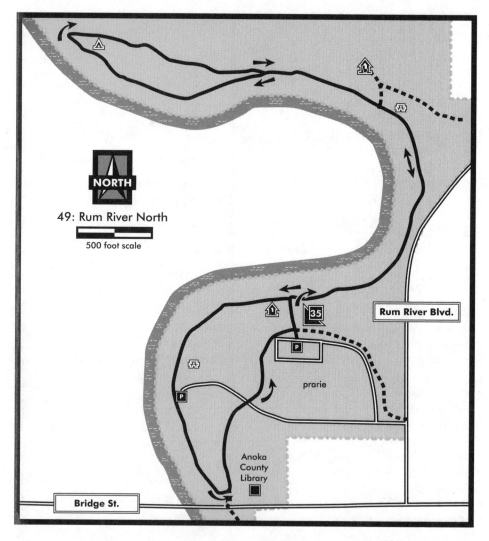

49: Rum River North

500 foot scale

Rum River Blvd.

prarie

Anoka
County
Library

Bridge St.

intersection, and take a right to follow along the river bank heading upstream of the Rum. You'll pass by a platform that overlooks the river presenting a nice water's-edge view up and down stream. The river is not too wide at this point and the banks are covered in foliage and trees overhanging right to the water.

The trail becomes crushed gravel shortly after leaving the center complex of picnic area and parking. The trail meanders through stands of oak and maple common to this area. Other hardwoods line the

bank above the river and along the trail for a few hundred yards until you reach an open meadow-like area on the right. Here you'll spy another picnic area and pavilion with several sets of tables. The river at this point flows along the base of a fairly steep embankment but always in close proximity to the trail.

On the river side of the trail where it opens to this meadow, you'll find sumac, oaks, and a few red pines. The trail then swings to the left and drops to very near the river's edge. Notice how the trees change from the upper hardwoods of oak and maple to the lower floodplain varieties of box elder and silver maple. These are fast growing trees of much softer wood than their upland neighbors.

Soon the trail splits; this is the intersection for the northern loop. Either fork brings you back to the main trail. Stick to the river's edge by taking the left fork. This trail clings to the river as it passes through a stand of silver maples. Soon you will come to another intersection to the right at the top of this loop. That trail spur leads a few yards out to the canoe camp and take-out site.

As you continue around the loop you move away from the river and soon come upon a marshy area past the trees on the left. Look for some water bird activity in this area in the spring and early summer. This trail loops back to the main trail and brings you back along the same route, which leads back to the starting T intersection up by the first pavilion.

Once you reach that T again, keep going straight to reach the southern half of the park. Laid out the same way as the northern section, the trail follows the river and loops at the end to bring you back through the park.

This trail seems to snake through the woods a bit more than does the northern section and the rolling nature of it as it dips and climbs the shallow hills makes

for a nice undulating walkway along the river. It comes out at a lower parking area and picnic ground. This is a very peaceful, pleasant area just north of the highway bridge crossing the Rum River in St. Francis.

The trail takes a hard turn to the left at the bridge and goes up to an access point next to the Anoka County Library. To return to the center parking area, head back through the parking lot and take the road out of the parking lot and up the hill. You will come to a trail intersection on the left. This winds through the woods and ends up back at the main pavilion.

A great way to enjoy this park would be to bring a picnic lunch and park at the southern lot. You could then take your lunch and stop over at the canoe take-out area at the extreme northern for a picnic before heading back down. Or you could leave your basket of goodies at the southern end and hike the entire loop before enjoying a picnic right along the riverbanks at the south end of the park. Either way, it's a good way to enjoy this short stretch of the Rum River.

NEARBY ACTIVITIES

Other hikes are farther north so your planning may include this hike at the start or end of a day's hiking these northern Twin Cities routes.

#50
Sakatah Lake
State Park

IN BRIEF
The Dakota tribe of Wahpekita Native Americans called this area "sakatah" or "singing hills." The area represents the transition zone between the "big woods" and more open southern Minnesota prairie.

DIRECTIONS
From Twin Cities, take Interstate 35 south to Faribault (Exit 55) then go 14 miles west of Faribault on Minnesota Highway 60. Turn right at the park entrance then take the next left to park near interpretive center.

DESCRIPTION
There are two trail systems to consider at Sakatah Lake State Park: the trails within the park, and the 39-mile Singing Hills Trail corridor that's part of the state's system of converted railroad bed trails. This particular corridor links the towns of Mankato and Faribault. Hoping to get the flavor of each, I've incorporated a hike that forms an irregular loop that encompasses both.

From the Center, hook up with the campground access trail that heads down to the lake via a 0.3-mile trail. At about 0.2 mile, this trail intersects one of the park's main hiking trails—the Oak Tree Trail or Utah u Can trail. This intersection is just before the final downhill path to the Singing Trail.

KEY AT-A-GLANCE INFORMATION
Length: 2.2 miles

Configuration: Two stacked loops

Difficulty: Easy to moderate; portions are level and easy, others make a moderate climb to a 100-foot change in elevation

Scenery: Big woods feeling with long view down very narrow corridor

Exposure: Mostly shade

Traffic: State trail busy with bike traffic in summer, snow machines in winter

Trail Surface: State trail is wide paved surface; within park are narrow, earthen trails

Hiking Time: 1–1½ hours

Season: All seasons; spring for birds, fall for colors, winter for skiing

Access: $4 daily vehicle permit, $20 annual state park permit

Maps: Available at park headquarters or at www.dnr.state.mn.us/parks_and_recreation/state_parks/sakatah_lake

Facilities: Interpretive Center, rest rooms, showers, drinking water

Special Comments: Hiking and lakeside/boating activities offer much for everyone

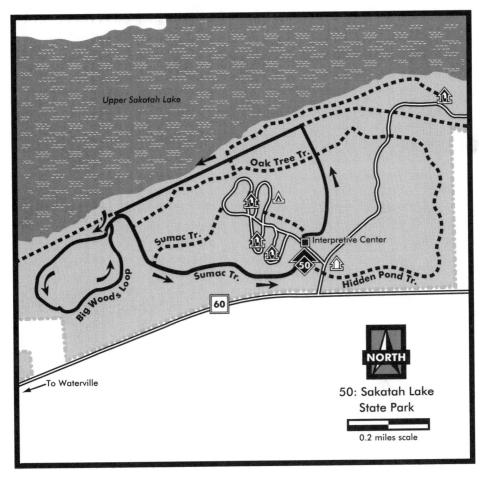

**50: Sakatah Lake
State Park**

0.2 miles scale

You can't miss the Singing Trail. This old railroad bed creates a wide, canopied corridor as it parallels the shores of Sakatah Lake—a widening in the Cannon River. Take a left (west) and head down the trail.

You hit the Wahpekita Trail 0.2 mile farther, which is a 0.6-mile trail along the lake shore to the fishing pier and lakeside picnic grounds.

By staying on the Singing Hills Trail, hikers can enjoy a paved, eight-foot-wide pathway that is as straight as an arrow—or at least straight as a former train track. Abandoned in the early 1970s, this used to be the route taken by the Chicago and Northwest Railroad.

However, to enjoy the park's trails you must leave the Singing Hills Trail at this intersection and take the trail to the left. This leads to the **T** intersection with the Oak Tree Trail. Take the Oat Tree Trail to the right. It parallels the railroad bed but allows you to continue hiking on trails within the park.

Continue on the Oak Tree Trail for about 0.3 mile to another **T** intersection, this time with the Sumac Trail. Take the Sumac Trail to the right and cross the bridge over the creek less than 0.1 mile farther. You will be at the beginning of the Big Woods Loop Trail just after you cross this bridge. Take the right fork and walk the loop counterclockwise.

The park has given this loop trail a Sioux name as well: "Tanka Canwitc." I've seen enough movies to convince me that "tanka" means 'big'. The Big Woods Loop is a 0.7-mile climb up and through the mature oaks and maples characteristics of the big woods forests that once covered this area of Minnesota. This area is what's called an ecotone—a transition zone between the Southern Oak Barrens and the Big Woods Landscape Regions.

Geologically speaking, this area was sculpted most recently by glacial activity about 14,000 years ago. A large glacial deposit, a moraine made up of rock and up to 400 feet deep, was laid down over the existing bedrock. As the glaciers receded, large chunks of ice were shoved into the ground. These melted forming the basins of lakes in the area, including Sakatah and Lower Sakatah lakes.

Coming down off the loop, you will need to re-trace your steps back over the bridge and continue south farther away from the lake. Ignore the first intersection, which is actually the west end of Oak Tree Trail. Instead, continue along the southerly trail for about 0.15 mile. You are now at the intersection with Sumac Trail.

Instead of taking the left trail, continue ahead to the south for about 0.5 mile. This is a hilly climb with lots of oak and map understory. The woodland you pass through developed after the Wisconsin ice age. This is the same look the forest had when the first non–Native American settlers began arriving.

You'll approach another trail junction toward the end of the Sumac Trail. This is lower Sumac Trail. It leads back to the main road and access to Hidden Pond Trail. Ignore it and continue that last bit back to your car.

NEARBY ACTIVITIES

The Singing Trail extends west 22 miles to Mankato or 14 miles east to Faribault.

#51
Sherburne NWR
(Prairie's Edge Trail)

3

169

51
Park
Entrance

4

Orrock

5   Zimmerman,
                          MN

IN BRIEF

This is designated as a driving tour but there is too much to see so take to foot and enjoy a hike through excellent marshes along the prairie's edge. This is a superb bird-watching tour.

DIRECTIONS

Go north from Minneapolis on US Highway 169 to Zimmerman. Continue 4 miles north to County Road 9. Go left (west) 5 miles to refuge headquarters (information on other hiking systems within the refuge is available at the headquarters). Continue past refuge office another 2 miles to CR 5. Turn left (south) and drive about 2 miles to entrance to Prairie's Edge Drive on left. Park in small lot immediately on your left about a quarter of a mile from the entrance near the observation station and a handicapped-accessible trail.

DESCRIPTION

While "Prairie's Edge" describes the overall topography and terrain character-istics of this hiking area, Marsh's Edge would seem a more appropriate name for the immediate and surrounding nat-ural experience one gets from hiking this area. Although this is called a driving trail, there is much too much to observe along these 7.3 miles to chance missing any of it by driving, even at 5–7 miles per hour. The entire marsh community is more easily viewed without the drone

KEY AT-A-GLANCE INFORMATION

Length: 7.3 miles

Configuration: Loop with two short side-spur options

Difficulty: Level, very easy

Scenery: Open meadows and marshes with a few scattered islands of trees

Exposure: Mostly full sun, some shade

Traffic: Occasional vehicle and bike traffic but probably not ever too crowded

Trail Surface: Hard-packed gravel roadway

Hiking Time: 2½–3 hours

Season: April through October

Access: No fee

Maps: Available in box inside entrance or at www.midwest.fws. gov/sherburne/prairie

Facilities: There are no facilities at this site

Special Comments: Use caution when sharing the road with vehicles

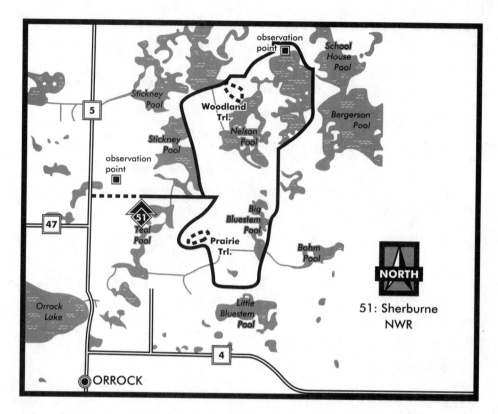

51: Sherburne NWR

of a car's engine or tires grinding over its gravel surface.

Sherburne National Wildlife Refuge (NWR) publishes a bird list featuring over 230 species common or transient to the refuge. If you are a birder and a hiker, this place will reward you several times over. Make sure you bring your binoculars on this hike!

Before starting, take a quick look from the observation deck, then head east along the entrance road. The first 0.75 mile brings you straight into the heart of the Sherburne NWR. About 0.5 mile from the observation area there is a small pond on the right. It's called Teal Pool. It and 23 other pools throughout the park have been enhanced from natural-occurring, uncontrolled pools and their water levels are regulated to create a number of different wetland types.

The prairie/marshland mix preserved in this park is a prime example of what these prairie-bordering areas were like as transition zones between the forested areas of the eastern US and those of the tall-grass prairies of Minnesota and beyond. Many of the wild critters and birds indigenous to this area today are the same species that were found here over 150 years ago—just as the settlers into this region found them. In all, the refuge covers over 30,000 acres in a mosaic of oak savanna, wetlands, and the big woods habitat.

The road around the Prairie's Edge directs visitors counterclockwise around the loop, so don't take the intersection you come to on your left near the end of this first straightaway road. Instead, go straight another 0.2 mile and follow the road as it turns sharply to the right. You are now on the loop that will continue for another 6 miles.

Teal Pool will be on your right as you climb a bit into the higher prairie country. As the road cuts back to the left there is a short side trail on the left, called the Prairie Trail. It's a short, 0.4-mile loop through typical tall-grass meadow and prairie vegetation. About 0.3 mile beyond the Prairie Trail, the road swings right again to lead through the first of many marshy areas. You will also cross over one of the many drainage canals used to regulate the water in all the pools throughout the refuge.

Crossing this marsh grass area, the trail cuts left again and passes along Little Bluestem Pool. An observation area at the middle point of the pool is a good area to try to spot some of the water birds and shore species that frequent the park. Using your binoculars, inspect the edges of the rushes right at the waterline for such species as little green herons and sora rails—otherwise very hard to spot against the backdrop of rushes.

A quarter mile past this lookout, the road turns north and for the next mile and a half cuts along the edge of several pools including the many ponds of Big Bluestem Pool on the left. You may have the best luck spotting critters by walking a few yards and then stopping for a few moments and studying any movements you see. Along this entire roadway are signs with black symbols representing songbirds and other wildlife that may be seen in the immediate vicinity.

About a half mile past the end of the Big Bluestem Pool, the road swings slightly to the right to pass between two of the refuge's biggest pools—Bergeson Pool on the right and Nelson Pool on the left. Bergeson is nearly a mile across. As the roadway heads north it comes right alongside Nelson Pool to skirt its shoreline for the next 0.7 mile or more.

The road turns northwest and then due west at the upper end of School House Pool. At the northwest tip of the pool is yet another observation area. If you look due south a few hundred yards, you should see large dead tree with an eagle's nest at its top. If there are too many people there to get a good view, don't worry, there is actually a closer viewing point farther along the trail, just after it makes a 90 degree turn to the left (south). A few hundred yards farther it starts to turn again. On the left is the pool and there should be a few thin spots in the bordering trees to get a good look at the nest.

The trail now turns to the southwest where you will come upon a sample of the woodlands associated with the oak savannah habitat. Look for songbirds in this area. Although a common nester in the park, I spotted my first rose-breasted grosbeak in this area during my hike. About 0.5 mile from the bend in the road where you viewed the eagle nest through the trees, there is another trail spur called the Woodland Trail. This 0.5-mile trail takes you through one of the woodland islands common to this oak savannah country.

The next 0.5 mile skirts along yet another pool, this one unnamed on the map. The trail then drops south again and passes Stickney Pool. The next 0.6 mile takes you right along its edge, too. By now you should be pretty good at spotting all the creatures hiding among the rushes.

The road comes to a **T** intersection. This is the end of the Prairie Edge Loop. A right takes you back to the first observation area and your car.

NEARBY ACTIVITIES

There are two other hiking trails within the Sherburne NWR. The Mahnomen Trails has about 2.6 miles of trails and the Blue Hill Trail offers a network of over 5 miles of trails. Both of these are north of the Prairie Edge trail system and offer more upland features and critters. These trails are especially good to take during the spring and fall migrations when the woodland songbirds are passing through.

You might also want to visit Ann Lake/Sand Dunes just a few miles south of the refuge.

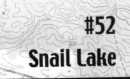

#52
Snail Lake

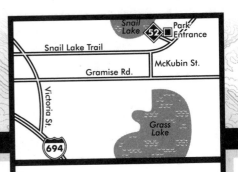

KEY AT-A-GLANCE INFORMATION

Length: 3.2 miles

Configuration: Barbells

Difficulty: Easy to moderate with a few steep areas

Scenery: Pleasantly woodsy with rolling hills, marshy transition zones, and open marsh in southern half

Exposure: Northern half is shaded; southern half exposed

Traffic: Eastern trail follows backyard boundary of homes, but southern marsh and northern woods areas offer solitude

Trail Surface: Paved throughout

Hiking Time: 1½–1¾ hours

Season: All seasons; snowshoeing is popular here in winter

Access: No fees

Maps: Intersections are marked, maps at www.co.ramsey.mn.us/parks/maps/snail_with_legend2

Facilities: Snail Lake has playground, picnic area, rest rooms, drinking water

Special Comments: Marsh areas are left in natural state, should be a good bird-watching park in spring and summer; it offers a good sense of northern woods even with houses visible right from trail and pedestrian underpasses beneath roadways

IN BRIEF

While Vadnais Lake gets top billing, a trail system south of Snail Lake is the notable hiking attraction in this multi-lake region of northeast St. Paul. The primitive marshy area right in the back yard of moderately-priced homes provides an appealing transition between the city and Minnesota's lakes and marshes.

DIRECTIONS

From Minneapolis, go North on Interstate 35 West to I-694. At Exit 43B (Victoria Street) go north (left) to Snail Lake Boulevard. From St. Paul, take I-35 East to I-694 and Exit 43B. Turn right (east) and go about 0.7 mile to park entrance on left (just past MacKubin Street).

DESCRIPTION

Snail Lake and Vadnais Lake share the spotlight for a multiple-lake regional park just outside the freeway loop around northern St. Paul. There are several trail options to consider, including a great sampler that begins in the parking lot of the Snail Lake Regional Park.

From the lot take the paved bike/hike trail that leads under Snail Lake Boulevard via a tunnel, or walk across the street from the entrance to hook up with the same trail. The paths immediately fork—take the right fork and head

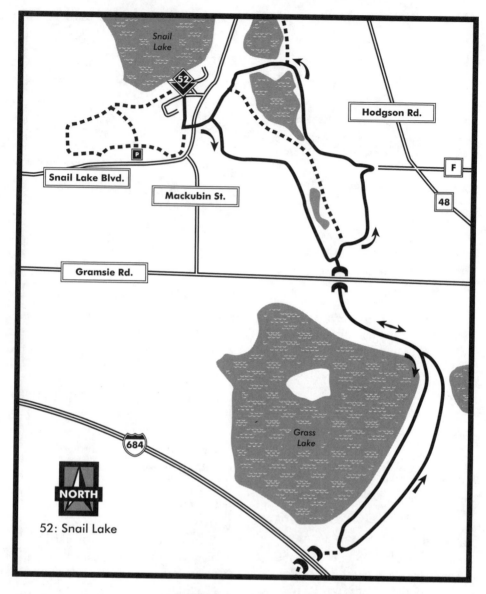

into the wooded area away from the marshy lowlands on your left. This trail heads slightly uphill through a scattering of oaks and maples. It's fairly open with older oaks sprinkled about. The path continues on to what first appears to be a knoll but as you walk deeper into the wooded area you learn that it's a knob on the side of the slope that drops down from the road and forms the sides of the basin that contains the marshy areas to the south.

The trail does become more hilly with red and white oaks becoming the dominant trees in the immediate area with a dense understory beneath. A few minor trails do spur off of this main trail. Their presence is made known only by modest hard-packed earthen paths that veer off as unannounced side trails. The ones on the left probably link up with the trails that cut down the center of the park.

Serpentine and hilly, the trail offers moderately easy hiking through dense but not imposing woodlands. About a quarter of the way down the first loop, you'll cross under a power line. There is a swath cut to the pond for a glimpse of what lies beyond the trees.

Like other parks surrounded by highways, this one has the sound of traffic woven into it. It's best to dwell not on the noise but on the fact that you can walk through trees rather than alongside fast-moving cars on a freeway.

As you near the southern end of the Snail Lake loop of trails you'll come through a short corridor of young aspen. As you come out of it you'll see Gramise Road in the background. A stand of cedar trees flanks the hill on the left overlooking a grassy meadow area through which the trail extends before going under the road to continue along the east side of Grass Lake. For those desiring only a short hike, keep on the paved path as it swings left away from the tunnel beneath Gramise, and follow the directions below for this 1.2-mile jaunt. Otherwise, head for the tunnel for the remaining 2 miles of the hike.

The trail forks shortly after the tunnel. Follow the hiking trail right alongside Grass Lake. At the bottom of the loop you'll come to the intersection with the bike trail. The bike path to the right joins up with a regional bike corridor, but you want to take a left and head back to the tunnel.

When you have returned to the pedestrian/bike underpass, turn right, and after about 80 yards the trail forks. The right fork heads to the east and follows the eastern side of the marsh while the left fork stays along the bike trail that cuts down the center of the park. Take the right fork for a slightly longer walk, and one that stays closer to the edge of the marshy area.

This pathway also follows the backyard property lines of houses that are adjacent to the trail. Aspen, box elder, some maples and hazel brush line this walkway that is about 40 feet from the marshy shoreline.

About three-fourths of the way around the marshy area, there are more islands and outcroppings of alders, willows, and shrub-like trees. Alders are like little birch trees as they have the same shaped leaves and catkins.

The marsh is long and narrow with cottonwoods at its northern end. More houses skirt the perimeter just before the trail turns around back to the start. There is another fork at the northeastern end of the lake that, if taken, leads you north to the intersection of the trail with County Road 96. There you are directed to more hiking along a regional trail. Otherwise, take the trail fork to the left. The trail swings back around into a hilly area before coming back down the back side of that small marsh you passed on your way in. You can take the underpass tunnel back to the parking lot.

NEARBY ACTIVITIES

There is a pathway around Vadnais Lake to the northeast, accessible by following Snail Lake Boulevard to the east. Other corridors like Vadnais from the north.

#53
Spring Lake Park Reserve
(Schaar's Bluff Trail)

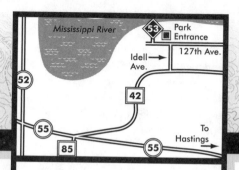

Mississippi River 53 Park Entrance

Idell Ave. → 127th Ave.

52

42

55 To Hastings

85 55

IN BRIEF

Truly a park that feels like northern Minnesota in its scenic bluff-line trails and woodlands. Spring Lake Park Reserve has incredible vistas of the Mississippi River—all captured along the Schaar's Bluff Trail.

DIRECTIONS

From Minneapolis/St. Paul, take US Highway 52 south to MN 55. Turn left (east) toward Hastings. Drive 4.5 miles to County Road 42, then turn left and go 1.8 miles to Idell Avenue. Take another left and follow road 1 mile to park entrance. Turn right into park and drive to parking lot at end of road.

DESCRIPTION

As well groomed and nicely developed as this park unit is, I was surprised to find such rustic, natural trail segments. Spring Lake Park has been called the "hidden jewel" of the Upper Mississippi. Like so many other hikes along the Mississippi corridor, the Schaar's Bluff trail system showcases the scenic bluff area of the Mississippi in a widening of the river called Spring Lake. The park is only a few miles upstream from the confluence of the St. Croix River.

Starting at the parking lot, take the trail that heads east (right) into the woods at the edge of the grassy extensions of the picnic and play areas. In fact, the first half mile of this trail appears to

KEY AT-A-GLANCE INFORMATION

Length: 2.9 miles

Configuration: Two loops

Difficulty: Easy; mostly level with a few gradual slopes; side trails require a little more careful footing

Scenery: Magnificent views of Spring Lake on the Mississippi with grand views of the river valley; expansive meadows rich in wildflowers in the summer

Exposure: Wooded areas are quite dense along bluff; full exposure on trails through open meadows

Traffic: Once trail levels in public area there are long, uncrowded stretches

Trail Surface: Mostly wide, 8-foot lanes with a few narrow game trail spurs, particularly on northern loop

Hiking Time: 1¼–2 hours

Season: All seasons; some trails groomed for cross-country skiing

Access: No fees

Maps: At park headquarters or at www.co.dakota.mn.us/parks/spring

Facilities: Fully developed day use park with picnic area, rest rooms, drinking water, playground

Special Comments: Take the time to enjoy the short spur trails

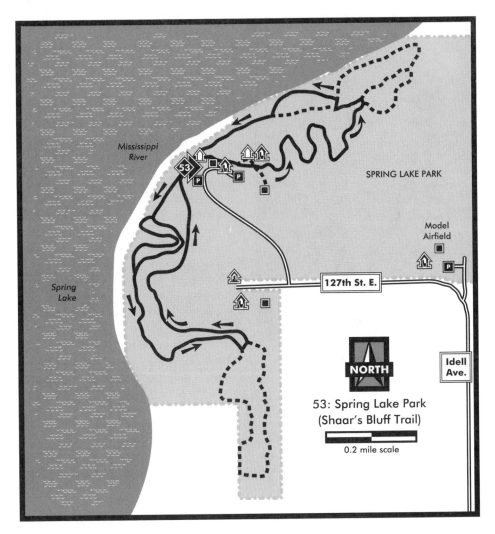

Mississippi
River

SPRING LAKE PARK

53

P

P

P

Model
Airfield

Spring
Lake

127th St. E.

NORTH

Idell
Ave.

53: Spring Lake Park
(Shaar's Bluff Trail)

0.2 mile scale

have been laid out by someone who couldn't decide whether to walk through the woods or along the open spaces. The trail does both. It's a wide, mowed avenue through basswood, oaks and ash. The trail snakes in and out of these woods twice before finally turning toward the top of the bluffs high above the river. The first part of this trail could be muddy after rains or during spring thaw. There are now red maples and red oaks mixed in with the other hardwoods.

At 0.57 mile from the trailhead the path intersects one of two short spur

trails. If you go right and take the 0.3-mile loop through the woods it will bring you back to the same intersection. This loop also opens up another 0.29-mile loop that brings you even closer to the bluff line before returning to the trail. These trails are unnamed but are well marked on the map with distances listed for each segment.

If you save these optional loops for another day, continue past the first inter-section and go a short distance (about 80 yards) to the next one. This is the 0.29-mile bluff trail described above. You can

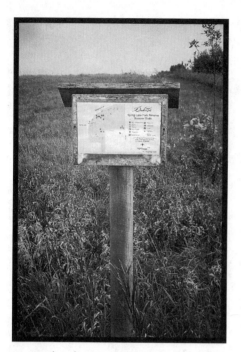

A typical trail sign at Spring Lake Park.

continue straight ahead but if you want to follow along the bluff, turn right, walk another few yards, then turn left to follow the bluff trail. This is a short 0.17 mile loop—one of the best in the park!

If there is ever a trail museum, this stretch should be in it as indicative of the small deer-and-game trails from antiquity that original settlers would have used to traverse this undeveloped land. Its narrow, earthen, bare footpath is worn into the forest floor. It is typical of the lacework of trails one expects to find woven through a birch-and-maple stand on the north shore. Occasionally a root snakes its way across your path and an exposed rock seems strategically placed smack dab in the middle of the pathway.

Its a quite a bit more rustic, less groomed, and not as fancy as the other trails in the park—and its far, far too short! I was enjoying the trail so much

that I had gone down half of it before I realized I had missed all the vistas overlooking the river and beyond. Several openings from the side of the trail award hikers with splendid views of the river below and the outstretched valley to the northwest.

Rejoin the main trail from the bluff line, turn right and continue back another 0.19 mile to the east end of the picnic shelter area.

There are wonderful, breathtaking vistas all along the edge of the park at this point. A carpet of lawn, seemingly held in place by stately oak trees, extends the entire length of this developed area. There is no trail, but if you continue along the edge of the bluff you eventually come to the lower half of the trail segment that loops out-and-back, first through more woodlands and then through patches of prairie at the western edge of the park.

About 0.16 mile south from the picnic shelter, there is a steep ravine cut from springs deep within the bluff itself. There are two trails from which to choose. The trail to the right cuts down into part of the ravine and back up the other side for a 0.3-mile segment. The left trail takes the high ground and pulls out into the edge of the meadowland to the east. Both of these two sections are less developed, and again a hiker can easily imagine and enjoy how trails have been developed over the centuries— from deer paths to mowed boulevards between the trees.

The two paths join and once again you will parallel the river before coming out onto patchwork sections of prairie between small islands and corridors of trees including a small stand of fine-needled white pine. Beyond is a farmstead—creating yet another image of bygone eras in this region.

The southern half of this loop drops down across the open, rolling hills of this grassland before swinging up toward the developed area of the park. The first leg is 0.41-mile long. It meets up with an optional 0.74-mile loop that drops down into the extreme southern portion of the park—away from the river.

Otherwise, the walking is casual from here on back. The trail continues on the loop that brought you along the park's southern portion.

This segment follows the gently rolling hills covered in meadow grasses that dominate the southern portions of the park. It winds along for 0.64 mile and reenters the picnic area by the parking lot.

NEARBY ACTIVITIES

Adjacent to this eastern section of the park is a separate airfield for remote controlled model airplanes. The western unit of Spring Lake Park has a double-circle, walk-through archery range. The entrance to each area is on the main road, left (east) to model airplanes, or right (west) to the outdoor archery range.

#54
Tamarack Nature Center

H-2
Park
Entrance
5
54
Otter Lake Rd.
Hammond Rd.
Exit
117

IN BRIEF

This one square mile patch of nature offers a short, easy hike through a marsh setting, typical of many of the forested regions of central Minnesota.

DIRECTIONS

Unmarked on many maps. Take Interstate 35 East north from St. Paul to County Road H-2 (about 1.7 miles north of Minnesota highway 96). Exit eastward (right) to Otter Lake Road. Turn south (right) and drive to park entrance (about 300 yards). Trailhead starts at far end of lot near interpretive center.

DESCRIPTION

For a compact natural area surrounded by freeways, Tamarack Nature Center offers a pleasant example of north woods diversity. The only thing missing at the Tamarack Nature Center—tamarack trees! Wildlife abounds and the setting takes you to the marshy alder bogs of northern Minnesota. While there are several alternate routes to choose within this small park, this hike passes through the heart of the park and is probably the quietest path.

Immediately behind the visitor center you'll see an eight-acre prairie restoration project. Prairie grasses and wildflowers dominate this otherwise open, flat field characteristic of the prairie meadows that once dominated this region.

The five-foot-wide paved pathway here is great for wheelchairs and

KEY AT-A-GLANCE INFORMATION

Length: 1.3 miles (up to 6.4 miles of trails available)

Configuration: Full circle loop from visitor center with many optional routes

Difficulty: Easy, mostly level

Scenery: Lots of birch, aspen surrounded by grasslands and alder marshes

Exposure: Mostly full sun, some shade

Traffic: Stay in center of park to avoid ambient highway noise; trails busier nearer the nature center

Trail Surface: Paved trails, earthen paths, and wooden walkways

Hiking Time: 45–60 minutes

Season: All seasons; skiing and snowshoeing popular in winter

Access: No fees, ample parking in lot at visitor center entrance

Maps: Available at visitor center or www.co.ramsey.mn.us/Parks/maps/tamarack

Facilities: Nature Center, rest rooms, drinking water

Special Comments: A haven for wildlife; the park offers good interpretive signage for the indigenous trees along interpretive route

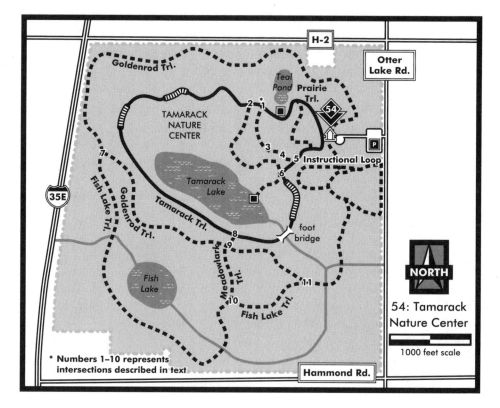

H-2

Otter Lake Rd.

Goldenrod Trl.

Teal Pond

Prairie Trl.

TAMARACK NATURE CENTER

2 1

54

3

4 5 **Instructional Loop**

7

6

35E

Fish Lake Trl.

Goldenrod Trl.

Tamarack Lake

Tamarack Trl.

8

foot bridge

9

Meadowlark Trl.

Fish Lake

NORTH

11

54: Tamarack Nature Center

10

Fish Lake Trl.

1000 feet scale

* **Numbers 1–10 represents intersections described in text**

Hammond Rd.

strollers, and basically makes a loop around the restoration project. You'll also begin the hike here. When ready, head right (north) along the Prairie Trail.

About 700 feet down the trail you'll come to a small wooded area of aspen and oak surrounding a smaller pond. This is Teal Pond and it offers a modest observation deck at the end of a very short spur trail. About 200 feet past that turn-out is Intersection 1, clearly marked on the left. The paved path sweeps left, but you want to right at the Intersection 1 marker and continue on around the side of Tamarack Lake. You'll come upon Intersection 2 a short distance later. This, too, goes through the wooded area bordering the restoration area but is more towards the marshy edges of Tamarack Lake. Again, stay to the right for a longer hike.

Now called the Tamarack Trail, it continues on through another small stand of woods and then back through more open grasses and islands of trees. It circles around another marshy area to the north before becoming a wooden footpath along the edge of yet another marshy area to the left. There are quite a few deer in this area (based on the many deer tracks). That and a sighting of four just beyond the wooden walkway in the middle of the day indicates that the deer are plentiful and not too shy with hikers.

At the northwest end of the park, the trail cuts south through a thick stand of alders and marsh grass. The alders are quite tall in this area creating a tunnel-like walk beneath their canopy. Once you've crossed this neck of marsh, you are facing a long, grass-covered hill which appears to be the highest elevation in the park. The trail turns to the left and passes beside the tree line growing along the edge of Tamarack Lake and the grass cover on the right.

At about 0.4 mile after coming out of the alders, you'll hit trail Intersection 8 and the Meadowlark Trail, opening up a number of hike alternatives as it goes southward and disappears over the ridge. Taking this trail will connect hikers up with Fish Lake Trail and channel them east about 0.7 mile back to the visitor center or out to the trails that follow along the park's western perimeter.

However, this hike continues along the edge of the lake for another 600 feet before re-entering the alder-thicketed marsh area at the southern end of the lake. There is a small foot bridge followed by an extensive section of wooden walkway. Both ends of the lake are good birding areas. This marshy area, while not totally appealing as a scenic feature, nevertheless is very representative of such vast marshy areas in Minnesota and elsewhere—and duly represented here to be appreciated on its own merits.

The trail comes out at Intersection 6. Turn right onto the stretch of paved trail, the interpretive loop, which circles back around the northern route to the visitor center. This and later sections are part of the interpretive loop that offers information on the trees you see en route. Head straight until you see the marker for Intersection 5. (The trails you see to the right are part of the instructional loop for cross-country skiers in the winter) and continue straight, back toward the visitor center and where you began.

Interestingly, the only tamarack trees I saw were growing outside the visitor center. There is a large one just south of the center's back side, right next to the trail. There's another along side the building. (For a great opportunity to walk among the tamarack, check out the hike listing for Tamarack Trail, page 197).

Nearby Activities
This park is only about fifteen minutes north of Vadnais-Snail Lake if you want more hiking adventures on your plate.

#55
Tamarack Trail, Lowry Nature Center/Carver Park Reserve

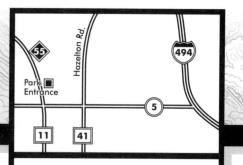

IN BRIEF

This trail meanders through all the represented ecosystems of the park—from oak forests to a watery network of lakes and marshes. The many interconnecting loop trails all feeding from the Lowry Nature Center provide for many short, but resource-rich hikes.

DIRECTIONS

Drive west on Interstate 494 to Minnesota Highway 5, then go west about 10 miles to Coomty Road 11. Turn right (north) 2 miles to entrance to Lowry Nature Center. Go to end of Nature Center and park.

DESCRIPTION

Carver Park Reserve covers over 3,000 acres, one-third of which are interconnecting lakes, marshes, and sloughs. Yet one of the most diverse areas of the park is represented in the area around the Lowry Nature Center located in the center of the park. This nature center has the distinction of being the first public environmental education center of its kind in the state. Its trail system offers a prime example of mixed woodland/marshland environment.

The park has an extensive trail system in the western section of the park via its horse-and-hiking trails that wind around three of the parks dozen large lakes. In addition, the eastern section offers over 7.4 miles of bike/hike trails that wind

KEY AT-A-GLANCE INFORMATION

Length: 1.5-mile interpretive loop connected to optional segments

Configuration: Loop

Difficulty: Very easy, mostly flat with several sections along boardwalks in the marsh areas

Scenery: Lots of vistas of open water and marsh

Exposure: Mostly sunny, some shade at beginning and end of hike

Traffic: If the nature center is busy expect the trails to be, too; otherwise there are enough trail spurs to find peace and quiet

Trail Surface: Mostly wide grassy trails; wooden walkways through marsh areas and tamarack trail loop

Hiking Time: 1–1½ hours

Season: All seasons

Access: $5 daily vehicle permit, $27 Patrons Annual Hennepin Parks permit

Maps: Available at nature center or at www.hennepinparks.org

Facilities: Nature center with rest rooms, drinking water

Special Comments: There is a great deal of natural history learn about in a small area; entire network can be explored in a day

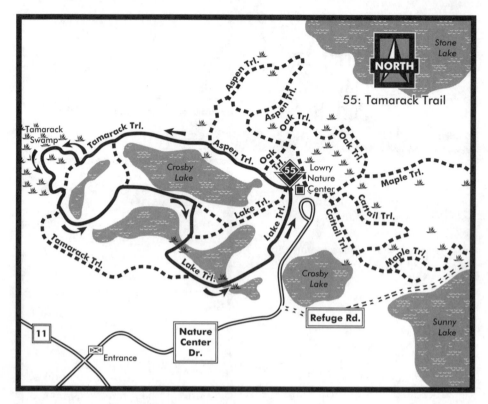

55: Tamarack Trail

between a half dozen more lakes. However, 5 or so miles of the interpretive trail system radiating out from the Lowry Nature Center in irregular loops are exclusively for hiking. While each segment is relatively short, they make up for it in natural features and amenities.

Beginning at the nature center (after you've spent time absorbing all the educational and informational displays and materials inside), take the Oak Trail toward the eastern end of Crosby Lake. This area is predominately oak with stands of maple and basswood. About 400 feet from the trailhead, the trail splits: Oak Trail veers to the right, and the Aspen Trail continues along the marsh grass and cattail shoreline of Crosby Lake. Take Aspen Trail at this point.

About 300 yards along the north shore of the lake, where the shoreline is especially marsh-like, the Aspen Trail cuts out away from the lake to the right and continues on its own loop and interconnections. The trail along the lake beyond the intersection with the Aspen Trail is the beginning of the Tamarack Trail. Continue straight ahead and stay next to the lake. Go another 400 yards to another trail intersection that cuts off to the left between Crosby Lake and a long, slender lake. That trail cuts back in a bit farther, but don't take it—there's a better route another couple hundred yards ahead.

Just as you are coming out of the woods, there is a trail to the right. This is the start of the 800-foot Tamarack Loop. I found this to be one of the most impressive features of this park. Tamaracks are quite common in northern Minnesota, less so around the Twin Cities. They look like other evergreens in the summer with their spire shaped growth and green needles. They loose their needles each fall just like the deciduous trees (oaks, maples, basswoods, ash, etc.) lose their leaves. They can appear to be a dead spruce tree to the unknowing eye.

The trail drops down into a dense marsh-like area and becomes a six-foot-wide boardwalk that snakes through islands of tamarack. Cattails and marsh grass at your fingertips without getting wet—that's what attracted me to this area. There are few marshes with such diversity and such accessibility. Usually you have to wait until winter when marshes freeze over to get this close. Here you can stroll along a wooden walkway right through the middle of this natural area at any time of the year with ease.

There is a jumble of deadfall and swamp brush, everything's a tangle—fallen just as Nature dictated. This is a very easy marsh to get to know because you can walk through it and observe up close instead of standing on its periphery and looking in. I've always thought tamarack stands had a prehistoric look about them.

Bring your binoculars and keep an eye out through out the tamaracks and grasses for redwing blackbirds and swamp sparrows, two of the more common birds in Minnesota's swamplands.

As you rejoin the Tamarack Trail on the western side of the lake, continue to the right. There's a picnic table on a small knoll. It faces the lake and the country to the east. The trail continues on along the high ground between Crosby Lake and the tamarack area before coming to a major intersection.

By mid-October the park is beginning to get ready for winter and snowmobiling. The hiking trail is dwarfed by a 30-foot-wide, grass mowed trail—a snowmobile highway. This trail cuts through the park and out onto the meadowlands to the left. This would be a good trail extension to take when wildflowers are in bloom.

Instead of continuing on the Tamarack Trail, I opted to follow this grassy superhighway mainly because it led back between more lakes as it cut its swath through the grassy area south of Crosby Lake. This trail connects back up with Tamarack after dropping south of the lake areas about a half mile farther along.

The north side of the trail provides open vistas cross Crosby Lake and the oaks beyond. The terrain in the Carver Park area is a result of deposits of the Wisconsin Age Des Moines glacial till. The hills and rolling topography are examples of the ground moraine created by that ice age. These land formations and the vegetation covering them is considered one of the best examples of an undeveloped complex of wetland/woodland/old field the Hennepin Parks system.

Archaeological evidence indicates that the lands in and around the park were used as hunting and fishing grounds—but not for village or dwelling sites.

The park supports a diverse population of wildlife: deer, Canada geese, swans, beaver, mink, gray and red fox, river otters, and a healthy population of song birds. Minnesota's seemingly ubiquitous red tailed hawk is a common inhabitant of the park as well. These lakes and adjoining meadows and woodlands create the perfect setting for attracting these and other critters.

Half way around the south end of Crosby Lake, the trail dips south and cuts into the woods surrounding the smaller lake. A small wooden footbridge crosses a narrow section of the lake, adding a rustic touch to the trail.

This is Lake Trail and it is the southernmost trail in this section that forms a connecting loop that goes out-and-back from the center. Here the oaks are a little more mature, and there are a few more pockets of marshes. Just beyond the footbridge is a interpretive sign that shares a bit of history about this particular area of the park.

In 1806, railroad tycoon James J. Hill, owner of the Great Northern Railroad, build a cut-away between Hopkins and Hutchinson—right through what is now this trail south of Crosby Lake. The tracks were removed in 1901 leaving this flat, straight section as the only reminder of events past.

The trail turns east and continues back through more trees bordering on a rolling meadow. Distant highway buzzing lets you know that you are still in an urban setting—but comfortably nestled in the environment of an active nature center. Another 300 yards and the trail crosses another modest footbridge. Although the trial winds in and out of the woods it remains flat and easy walking. Look for woodpeckers and chickadees in this section of the park. The trail continues on for about 400 yards to the hub of the trails at the Lowry Nature Center.

NEARBY ACTIVITIES

The Grimm Farm/Parley Lake area features both historic and natural amenities of this park. The Wendelin Grimm Farm was a 137-acre tract, and dates back to 1857. Grimm immigrated to Minnesota that year and spent the next few years developing a winter-hardy strain of alfalfa—the first ever developed in the United States. It was a significant leap toward the development of the dairy industry in the upper Midwest.

IN BRIEF

This is a small neighborhood park with a modest lake and pleasant oak stands to hike though. It's a short trail but has a more remote flavor once you get back into the hilly woods.

DIRECTIONS

Drive north on US Highway 52 (Lafayette Freeway), to Butler Avenue. Turn left and drive to Stassen Lane. Turn left into the park and stop at first parking lot on the right.

DESCRIPTION

The Thompson County hiking trail cuts several paths through this tiny chuck of big woods tucked in between freeway and houses on St. Paul's south side. Entering the park the impression is one of a country wayside next to a very small lake. For the most part, that's exactly right.

The hiking trail, in fact, begins at the parking lot and follows the paved pathway around the front of the information center. The path heads down to the small pond-like body of water called Thompson Lake. Turn right at the intersection, and follow the path, which is paved around the developed half of the lake. Just after a footbridge over the creek at the northern end of the lake, the path turns into a dense, crushed gravel path about five feet wide. The path continues around the lake and is flanked by sumac

KEY AT-A-GLANCE INFORMATION

Length: 1.4 miles

Configuration: Figure eight

Difficulty: Easy; rolling pathway with some steep inclines, also paved, smooth paths around lake

Scenery: Pleasantly woodsy with rolling hills

Exposure: Lake is sunny, but rest of hike is shaded

Traffic: Neighborhood park, modest usage

Trail Surface: Trail around developed side of lake is paved, the rest is hard pack

Hiking Time: 1 hour

Season: All seasons; especially busy in winter due to lighted ski trails

Access: No fees

Maps: Available from Dakota County or at www.co.dakota.mn.us/parks/thompson

Facilities: Picnic pavilion, rest room, playground, telephone

Special Comments: One of several regional corridor trails leads off from the 1-mile looped trail; it heads south along US 169 but does not connect to another trail at this time

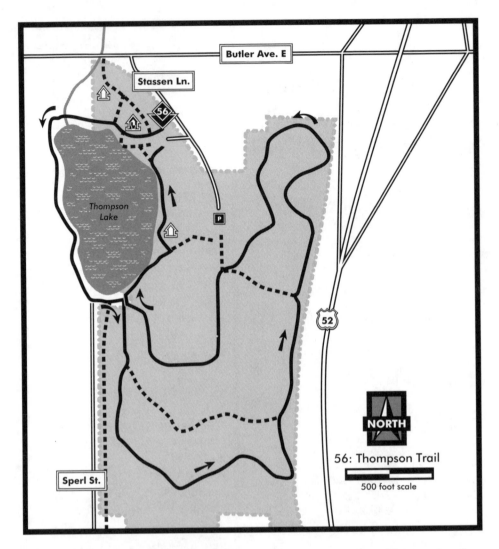

Stassen Ln.

56

Thompson
Lake

P

52

NORTH

56: Thompson Trail

500 foot scale

Sperl St.

on the shore side and a buffer zone of
grasses between the park and the adjoining neighborhood on the right.

Although very small (the entire park is
only 57 acres), the lake was bustling with
waterfowl activity the day I was there.
Mallards, songbirds (mostly warblers),
and even an egret took their collective
places along the little nicks in the otherwise even shoreline of the oval lake.

The trail continues south into woods
and patchy open areas. At the bottom of
this lake loop, you'll see a trail heading

right, a continuation of the gravel trail.
The first turn to the right is a continuation of the paved trail out of the park.
Stay on the main route and take the second grass trail that angles up a modest
grassy knoll and heads into the island of
trees ahead.

In this section you have a number of
options to create hikes of varying length.
For our purposes, we'll follow the
perimeter of this trail system to create a
1-mile loop. Continue down the trail
and ignore the path heading off to your

left—this will be where you return in a little while. Shortly after this intersection you'll come to a fork. The path to the left goes about 0.2 mile to intersect the larger loop trail. Stay to the right, however, and follow the loop along the southern half of the park.

This southern part of the park, like the rest of the wooded area, features abundant oaks and maples. Its topography and tree cover is typical of most of this area before development leveled off or filled in the natural wooded areas. The hilliness is reminiscent of glacial deposited kames and kettle areas nearby. In fact it is part of the St. Croix glacial moraine.

The loop cuts across the bottom third of the park then hits and parallels US Highway 52. The trail returns north, and in 90 yards intersects with the trail that leads back to the fork you passed earlier. The trail approaches another intersection on the left 200 yards farther along. You can take a short jaunt down this path to reach one of the highest points

in the park. Return to the main trail, heading north to enjoy another 0.43-mile loop that encircles the northern-most end of the park.

More oaks and upland understory are common throughout this area. The trail does move away from the freeway slightly before it circles around to come out at the end of the small parking lot at the end of the park entrance road. Follow the trail to the left and it will come out at the southern end of the lake. Take another right and follow the lakeshore back to the starting point at the parking lot.

NEARBY ACTIVITIES

The Mississippi River is a few miles to the east. A segment of the Mississippi Trail can be accessed for a short hike along the river by turning right (east) on Butler after exiting the park, cross Concord Street (CR 156) to river. There are turn-outs along the roadway and a few parking areas along the trail.

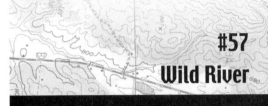

#57
Wild River

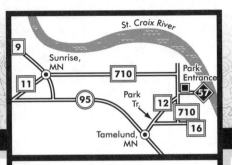

IN BRIEF

One of several state parks along the upper St. Croix River, Wild River offers a pleasant walk along its banks. Forests regenerated after decades of lumber harvesting are now mature stands of oaks and maples. Together the river and forest offer many of the natural amenities for which Minnesota parks are renowned.

DIRECTIONS

From Minneapolis take Interstate 35 West north to Minnesota Highway 95 in North Branch. Take MN 95 right (east) to County Road 12 in Almelund. Turn left (north) and go 3 miles to park entrance. Drive into park and take second major right, and follow sign to canoe rental/launch area. Park in the lot to the left of the canoe rental shed.

DESCRIPTION

Always a great river upon which to paddle, the St. Croix is equally rewarding from a hiker's perspective—St. Croix Wild River State Park offers a scenic river walk coupled with a hike through dense stands of Minnesota hardwoods.

This hike begins at the edge of the river, near the canoe rental site. At the turnaround, head south along the trail, which is marked several ways: Amik's Pond Loop, River Trail, and Deer Creek. All follow the same path from the trailhead sign at the edge of the road.

KEY AT-A-GLANCE INFORMATION

Length: 4.6 miles

Configuration: Loop

Difficulty: Easy; level with only a few inclines, some sandy areas by river

Scenery: The St. Croix Valley at its finest; river is in view for about half this hike

Exposure: Full shade except for meadow crossings

Traffic: Little along the river, expect campground and picnic areas to be utilized on weekends; boat ramps are popular

Trail Surface: About 40% paved trail; 60% earthen or mowed grass with some sandy areas

Hiking Time: 2–2½ hours

Season: All seasons; winter ski trails

Access: $5 daily vehicle permit, $20 annual state park permit

Maps: Available at park headquarters or at www.dnr.state.mn.us/parks_and_recreation/state_parks/wild_river/

Facilities: Campground, picnic area, rest rooms, showers, drinking water, canoe rental, boat launch

Special Comments: Expect to see lots of canoes on the river; good park to stop for a hike while canoeing

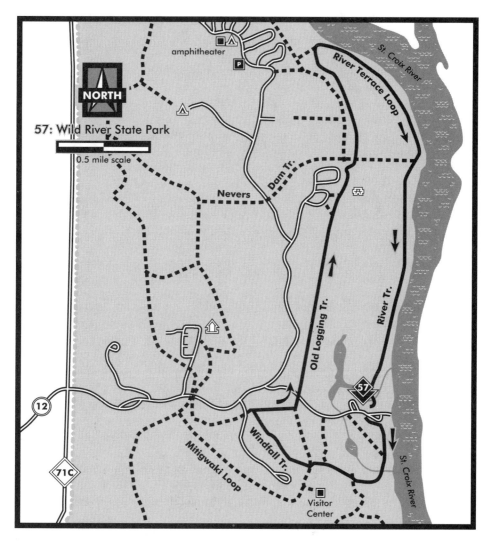

NORTH

57: Wild River State Park

0.5 mile scale

amphitheater

Nevers

Dam Tr.

River Terrace Loop

St. Croix River

Old Logging Tr.

River Tr.

57

12

71C

Mitigwaki Loop

Windfall Tr.

St. Croix River

Visitor Center

The trail is a six-foot, mowed, earthen path that follows the river a little beyond 0.2 mile before turning inland and upland. At 0.2 mile there is a spur to the right, the Amik Pond Loop turn-off. Stay to the left along the river for a few more yards before the main trail does turn to the right. You will leave the cover of ash and willow and head toward a stand of birch at the back edge of a meadow (check for deer in the early morning). You will then come to a T in the trail. The left branch of the T turns

south and becomes the Deer Creek Trail—also a horse trail. Stay to the right and continue onward around the southern end of Amik Pond. This area, as in the rest of the park, is alive with birds. Expect to see eastern pewees, mourning doves, Baltimore orioles, and warblers along this trail. For the next 0.2 mile you should also notice signage and interpretive points along this portion of the Amik Pond Interpretive Trail.

At the next intersection, the Amik Pond Trail spur goes right; stay left to

follow the Windfall Trail, another interpretive trail. You'll come upon a sign
leading you to the Old Logging Trail
and then the Old Logging Trail itself.
The trail climbs a bit, past a thick understory of ferns, ash, and oak saplings.

At the intersection of this wide, paved
trail, hang a left and go about 100 yards
to the remaining section of the Windfall
Trail. Take this trail to the right to continue the loop. You will pass through a
mature stand of oaks, ash, and birch—a
stately forest of older trees—a grand
sampling of some of Minnesota's noble
hardwoods.

About half way along this section
you'll come to a turnout on your left
with a bench and a strange, wood, table-
like contraption. It's a tree-finder and
identifier. It's pretty easy to figure out:
windows contain descriptions and illus-
trations of some of the major tree species
in the area (ironwood, basswood, oak,
etc.). Once you center the information
in the window, two sights line up that
allow you to find that tree in the cluster
growing around the tree finder. Sight
through the eyehole; check out the tree
that aligns with the V notch in the other
end and you've located the tree highlighted in the information window.

When you come to signpost marked
4 you have intersected the Mitigwaki
Trail, a paved trail that you want to take
to the right for 0.2 mile to rejoin the
Old Loggers Trail. You'll come to a T, at
which point you'll take a left to head
north. You'll soon cross a park road, but
keep going straight—into the heart of
the forest.

Up to now you've sampled the southern half of the park's hiking trails—to
the south and west, horse trails prevail.
However, the Old Logging Trail is a
wide avenue through a mature stand of
upland hardwoods. For the next mile

you'll experience a peaceful walk
through the upland woods of near-
northern Minnesota.

While hiking along this section, imagine loggers felling trees, trimming them,
and loading trunks onto large wagons
that drove up and down such roads.
Much of the logging was done in winter
when roads were solid and underbrush
was at a minimum. This was a significant
logging region and many roads like this
one were major arteries for getting the
lumber to the rivers for the float south
to saw mills on the St. Croix River.

After a mile, the trail opens onto the
developed picnic area. Several facilities
are available here including drinking
water, rest rooms, pavilion, and BBQ
pits. At the far end of the pavilion turn
right (east) onto the Nevers Dam Trail.
Almost immediately there is a cut to the
left off of the Nevers Dam Trail. This is
the River Terrace Loop, a 1-mile trail
that meets up with the St. Croix at 0.5
mile and then swings south (to the right)
along the river and back to the Nevers
Dam Site. Unless you want to cut off 1
mile of hiking to get to the Nevers Dam
Site (only 0.2 mile to the river), take the
River Terrace Loop to the left.

At the top of the River Terrace Loop
is a trail to the left called the Trillium
Trail. This trail heads northwest toward
the northern corner of the park where it
meets up with the Sunrise Trail and
actually continues upstream along the St.
Croix to another park unit section on
the Sunrise River. There's also a long
staircase that leads to the campground.
Save this hike for another day and continue around the loop to the right and
back toward the river.

The trail follows the river for 0.5 mile
before coming to the Nevers Dam Site.
There an interpretive sign will tell you
about this dam which was built to hold

back logs awaiting processing at the lumber mills downstream at Stillwater. This dam, built in 1889, was in operation until 1954. Before the dam was built huge log jams plugged the river for weeks costing lumber companies a lot of money in time and damaged or destroyed logs. In 1886 a massive log jam—containing enough timber to build 15,000 houses—blocked the river in this section for over six weeks! Over 100 logging camps used the St. Croix to move their timber south.

From the observation deck at the dam site, the trail spur heads back toward the picnic area. You want to take the trail leading off to the left as you face uphill and away from the river. This continues your river hike, and the trail now becomes the River Trail.

The trail follows the lowlands of the St. Croix, sometimes crossing sandbars that turn the trail into a brush-covered beach in spots. It stays close to the river for all of its 1.2-mile length back to the turnaround at the canoe rental site. About half way along the trail, a bench is conveniently placed atop the bank. It's a pleasant place to rest and enjoy the slow-flowing St. Croix.

At about 0.9 mile you will come to a canoe campsite directly off the trail to the right. After 20 yards another trail heads back into the woods on the right. This is a walk-in backpacker's campsite accessible from the canoe rental parking lot. It's a spacious, shaded campsite with picnic table, fire ring, primitive latrine, and wonderfully flat and smooth tent spaces. A great way to enjoy this hike is to come in the night before, camp here, and start out on the trail bright and early the next morning. You are only 0.3 mile from the start of the trail at this point.

From the campsites, the trail veers away from the river to go around a slough on the left. It then crosses over the slough via a foot bridge and comes out onto a lane about 100 yards from the canoe rental complex (road turnaround, parking lot, rest room, picnic table and boat access to the river). At the canoe rental shed, take a right back to the parking lot to complete this hike.

NEARBY ACTIVITIES

Northern section of the park includes the Sunrise River, another popular canoeing route. Not too much farther south is William O'Brien State Park.

#58
William O'Brien State Park (Upper Park Trail)

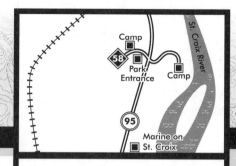

IN BRIEF

Besides its natural beauty and the St. Croix River, the big appeal of William O'Brien State Park is its proximity to the Twin Cities. There is a nice hiking loop along the river's edge in the lower park complex but a hiker really gets a workout exploring all the loops and side trails in the network of the upper park.

DIRECTIONS

From St. Paul drive north on Interstate 694 to US Highway 61 in Delwood. Turn right (east) onto Minnesota 96 and drive east to for about 9 miles to the intersection at the St. Croix River with MN 95. Turn left (north) and follow the road for another 9 miles through Marine-on-St. Croix to park entrance on left. Take park road to T intersection, turn left, then make an immediate right into Interpretive Center parking lot.

DESCRIPTION

This hike begins at the Interpretive Center and is aptly named the Upper Park Trail. Geologically speaking, the St. Croix Valley was cut by glaciers over 10,000 years ago. Remnants of that action are evident by the river though the deep gorges cut into the sandstone and lava-deposited rock. Upland, evidence of the glaciers includes rolling hills, potholes, and boulders of various sizes strewn throughout the forests and meadows. All of these upland clues are visible along this trail.

KEY AT-A-GLANCE INFORMATION

Length: 4.6 miles

Configuration: Loop

Difficulty: Easy; with gradual elevation changes

Scenery: Uplands, away from river, but large meadows with wildflowers, mature stands of hardwoods, expansive marsh area

Exposure: Mostly full sun, some shade

Traffic: Popular park, but most activity occurs down by the river

Trail Surface: Some mowed grass, other earthen pathway

Hiking Time: 2–3 hours

Season: All seasons

Access: $4 daily vehicle permit, $20 annual regional park permit

Maps: Available at park headquarters or at www.dnr.state.mn.us/parks_and_recreation/state_parks/william_obrien/

Facilities: No facilities in upper park beyond interpretive center's rest rooms; drinking water, campground amenities in lower park

Special Comments: This part of the park is much less seen by most visitors; wildflowers bloom in profusion during summer, particularly in meadows near Interpretive Center

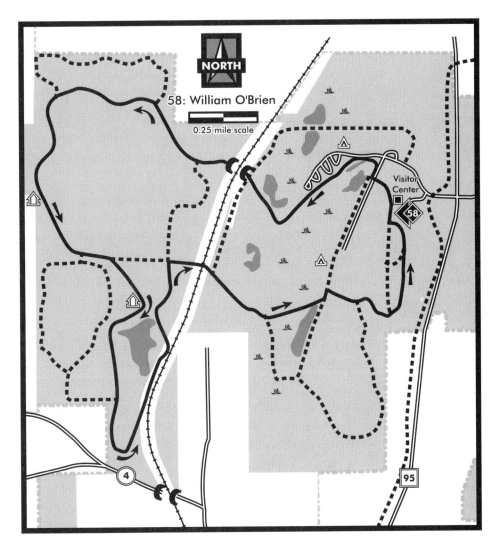

58: William O'Brien

0.25 mile scale

NORTH

Visitor Center

From the center head out behind the building to the trailhead sign. Carry a map with you as each trail intersection is numbered for easy orientation. The spur from the Interpretive Center intersects with a broad trail a couple hundred yard past the center. Take a right to get onto the main loop. You will see the maintenance building ahead of you and the trail will swing to the left across a park road. This intersection with the park road is Intersection 1.

The upper park area contains a mix of hardwoods and meadows. The first part

of the trail meanders through box elders and a mixed conifer forest of spruce and pine.

After you cross the road turn right and continue behind the campgrounds; you are skirting a bog-like area on the left. Its rushes indicate a moist, soggy soil. Box elder, ironwood, and basswood trees also hint at a lowland type of ecosystem common to this area. As the trail rises in elevation, white pines come into view and you will pass several trail spurs leading back to the campground on the right. This higher elevation transition continues along the trail as you pass sumac, cedar, and oak trees.

Soon after passing the campground be on the watch for a monstrous basswood on the right. Its big, heart-shaped leaves and gigantic size will be a give-away. These trees are also called lindens, particularly when used in landscaping. Be careful while looking up at this giant, the trail is flanked with a thick growth of poison ivy in this section.

Just before Intersection 2, at a sharp bend in the trail to the right, you'll come through a corridor of oak and ironwood. There is a bench right at the bend in the trail. The trees in the marshy area to the right are all dead. At first one would think the marshy area developed some time after the trees were established and eventually drowned them out. A closer inspection of the tree's lower trunk shows clear signs of charring from a fire.

An interpretive sign later in the trail does indicate that a controlled burn took place here. These are used to reduce excessive understory, clean up accumulated deadfall, and encourage new growth. Some seeds need heat to break their tough seed coats so a brush fire oftentimes is the only way they can germinate. New sprouts from regenerated plants attract wildlife into an area as well. It's good use of fire for keeping areas healthy.

The trail passes through this boggy area and comes to major Intersection 3 right before a foot tunnel under the railroad tracks. You could take either a left or right to make this a much shorter walk or, as this hike does, continue on under the tracks (follow the Hiking Club Trail sign) and head for Intersection 4 as shown on the map.

At Intersection 4 you will have hiked about 1.6 miles, and once again have the option to alter the hike by heading south to parallel the train tracks. Otherwise, keep going straight toward Intersection 5 as this brings you into higher country. The elevation at the bog was about 840 feet. You'll climb to about 1020 feet if you stay on this trail and continue along the main route between Intersections 5 and 8. It crosses the face of three small ravines and skirts the northwestern most parts of the park. About halfway along this loop you'll come to a shelter and toilet. There is also a trail to the left that cuts back through the middle of this particular loop that does not appear on the maps. It may be only a winter ski trail but it can be hiked and it comes out just before the Intersection 5.

After looping around the northern portion of upper woodlands and meadows, the trail comes to Intersection 8; the trail to the right leads to a fire break loop. Stay on the main trail and continue on to Intersection 9. To shorten the hike by a mile, continue straight to Intersection 11. Otherwise head right (south) to follow a 1.5-mile loop that encompasses one of the few lakes in this section. The trail reaches its southern terminus and heads north again, eventually descending a hill into a meadow area. Just before the Intersection 11 there is a diagonal spur to the right. It's just a shortcut to the right; go ahead and take it and turn right at the next intersection, heading east.

Go up and over the railroad tracks to Intersection 12. A word of caution: these are active tracks, but there are no warning flashers, be sure to watch for approaching trains. Continue past Intersection 12 for 0.3 mile to Intersection 13. Along the way, you'll see a marshy area sprawled out before you. It's a pleasant vista and gives you a sense how the marshy areas integrate with the woods.

You will cross what appears to be a causeway, a raised trail bed across the wet, boggy area. I would expect to see an occasional water bird in this area, perhaps more so during spring and fall migration. There are plenty of song birds in this park including woodpeckers, bluebirds, orioles, herons, and a variety of warblers.

Bird-watchers may want to turn right at Intersection 13 and hike an extra 0.6-mile loop to take in the small pond just south of here. Otherwise, continue east to Intersection 17.

There are two distinct ridges that run north and south in this upper park. One is at the western end of the bog and is the site of the railroad bed. The other is along the trails just to the west of the visitor center. These two ridges contain the marshy area in the middle. You can really see this defined ridge line as you walk along the trail from Intersections 13 to 17.

Turn left at Intersection 17, then a right shortly thereafter. This brings you up and over this wooded ridge. It's a rise in elevation of about 50 feet. You'll pass under mature stands of oak and basswood. The trail opens onto a meadow, another small section of trees and yet another meadow before coming to Intersection 16. Keep to the left at this junction as you head through a stand of maples and basswood (lots of poison ivy again, too).

The trail intersects with an unmarked trail that goes off to the left. Don't take this unmarked trail; stay on the straight course that leads you out onto the prairie-like meadow before you. The Interpretive Center and the parking lot are ahead about 0.2 mile. The walk through this prairie is particularly enjoyable in mid summer when all the wildflowers are in bloom. If you bring a wildflower book, you could spend hours identifying all the species in bloom.

NEARBY ACTIVITIES

All the river activity is in the lower part of the park. There is a hiking trail along the river's edge can give you an additional 1.5 miles for the day. Interstate Park is about 15 miles north on Minnesota Highway 95.

#59
Willow River, Wisconsin

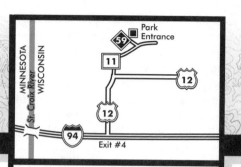

IN BRIEF

This trail and surrounding park surely deserve the title "hidden gem." Its attractiveness as a geological and culturally rich park is surpassed only by one of the most impressive waterfalls in this part of the state.

DIRECTIONS

From the Twin Cities take Interstate 94 to the marked exit for Willow River State Park at Mile 4 in Wisconsin. Head north on US highway 12 to County Road 42. Turn left onto CR U and go about 1.5 miles to the park entrance. Park immediately behind the park office.

DESCRIPTION

All the trails in the 3,000-plus acre Willow River State Park are designated by name—and by color. Colored posts along the route and at intersections help orient hikers as to what route you are on or intersecting. Head down the mowed spur trail at the northern end of the parking lot to reach the trailhead.

At the T intersection you join the Pioneer Trail (yellow). Take the trail to the right towards the Grave Sites and Willow Falls Trail (blue) as indicated by the signs at the trailhead. The Willow Falls Trail appears as wagon path, replete with ruts and a grassy, mounded center. Aspen and oak flank the left side of the trail, an open meadow extends to the right.

KEY AT-A-GLANCE INFORMATION

Length: 4.4 miles

Configuration: Loop with one-out-and-back spur

Difficulty: Easy to moderate, but with steep slopes to/from river

Scenery: Waterfall is impressive, lowlands by river and upland hardwoods pleasantly typical for region

Exposure: Sections of shade and sun throughout trail's course

Traffic: Any trail connecting to the waterfall trail will be popular

Trail Surface: Earthen, some gravel, and some parts muddy

Hiking Time: 2–3 hours, plus time to stop at the waterfall

Season: All seasons; some steep trails may be impassable in winter

Access: $5 daily Wisconsin residents, $7 out-of-state; $18 annual pass for Wisconsin residents, $25 out-of-state

Maps: Available at park headquarters or at www.pressenter.com/~thofern/

Facilities: Rest rooms, campground, drinking water, nature center, beach, boat launch

Special Comments: Plan to spend some time at the falls and bring your camera

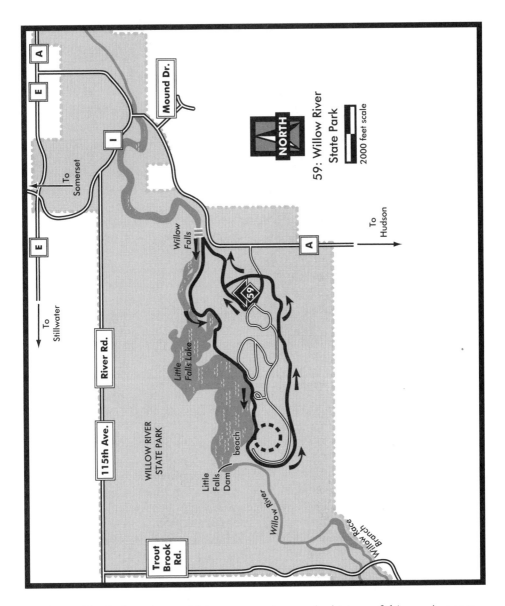

59: Willow River State Park

NORTH

2000 feet scale

To Somerset

To Stillwater

To Hudson

Mound Dr.

Willow Falls

Little Falls Lake

River Rd.

115th Ave.

Trout Brook Rd.

WILLOW RIVER STATE PARK

Little Falls Dam

beach

Willow River

Willow Race Branch

The trail leads down into a thick understory dominated by prickly ash. Soon basswoods and oaks, and an island of cedar trees will come into view. Five hundred feet down this trail you'll pass a small fenced section of grass that is labeled the William Scott Grave Site. The Scotts settled this area in 1849.

There is little detail about the Scotts' plight, however there is much informa-

tion on the history of this area in general. Prehistoric settlers in the Woodland Period practiced burying their dead in earthen mounds, many of which can still be found in the St. Croix River area nearby. Chippewa and Sioux shared this land—as enemies. Many wars broke out over the wild rice lakes in the area. One battle of record took place at the mouth of the Willow River in 1785.

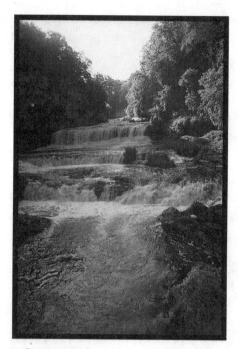
Willow River Falls.

the forest floor. It's more like a dried creek bed than a hiking trail. It's a continuous steep drop that winds down to the river. At the river bank you'll come to another T intersection. This is the Willow Falls Trail (blue). Ahead of you, through the trees, will be your first glimpse of a clear, trout-rich stream.

The falls are to the right, about 350 yards down the trail. Your ears will tell you what direction to follow. The falls are a series of cascading steps which send the roar of the water falling over rock down the valley. There is a footbridge at the base of the falls that provides a continuous viewing point across the river up- and downstream. A viewing platform just before the bridge offers a great place to rest and to enjoy the sounds of birds and cascading water.

The cut in the rocks through which the Willow River flows before tumbling down the rocky shelves was the site of a dam back in the wheat producing era.

The dam was one of several built by Christian Burkhardt, a German immigrant who helped develop the area's wheat industry. Influenced by hydroelectric power plants on a visit to Germany in the late 1800s, he built several power plants in the area. Eventually Northern States Power (NSP) purchased these power plants and when lightning damaged one of the plants in 1963 NSP decided it was no longer profitable to maintain the plants. In 1967 negotiations between NSP and the Wisconsin Conservation Commission created this park. The dam that was built in the gap between the two bluffs was removed in 1992.

The best time to visit the falls (which face south) for photo opportunities is in mid-afternoon when the sun swings across the valley and lights the face of the falls from the front.

Early white explorers included French, British and American frontiersmen and traders.

The proximity to the St. Croix (the Willow River joins the St. Croix a few miles to the west at the town of Hudson, Wisconsin) made this area prime for wheat and lumber: two commodities that relied on the river for transport and commerce.

Past the grave site, the trail continues on for about 300 yards where it comes to an intersection marked with a blue post. This is the trail that leads down to the river and Willow Falls. Take a left here. The right spur heads to an overlook of the falls another 300 yards farther along the bluff.

The blue trail swings steeply down into the thick of the woods, under a canopy of oaks, basswoods, and ironwoods. The trail is a wide, deep cut into

Across the bridge from the falls a trail continues up to two other overlooks and a series of looped trails on the other bluff. This hike, however, backtracks from the falls back to the T intersection at the base of the hill. This time, keep going straight along the Willow Falls Trail (blue) and continue the hike downstream.

The Willow Falls Trail is a little over 0.9-mile long and follows the course of the river. However, you won't see the river again until you are about halfway down the trail. Burr oaks, maples, and lots of poison ivy line both sides of the corridor through the trees. Just as the trail turns from packed earth and grass to gravel, check out the gigantic cottonwoods on the left. These are stately specimens.

The trail swings away from river to go around a slough. Check it out in early morning for deer or shorebirds such as egrets and great blue herons. The trail continues to swing left and climb as it rounds a section of the lake near the park's campgrounds. Here the Willow Falls Trail (blue) officially ends. Follow the campground roads keeping to the right until you come to the far end of the grounds near the campground rest rooms. There you can catch the trail that heads past the boat launch and the beach. The trail is now called the Little Falls Trail (green).

Just beyond the bathhouse the trail spurs to the right out to the dam for a nice side trip off the bigger trail loop. Back at the bathhouse, from the dam, take a right and continue on about 300 yards and cross the park road. You'll come to an intersection with the Trout Brook Trail (purple). Like the dam trail, this is another short loop along the river which adds a mile to the hike.

At the Trout Brook Trail (purple) intersection, go left along the Oak Ridge Trail (brown). This section is a mile-long stretch through some of the park's high country and stands of oaks. The Oak Ridge Trail intersects at 1 mile with the White Tail Trail (red). The Little Falls Trail. (Note: maps available at the park name this segment as the "Little Falls Trail"; however, the park tabloid, also available at the park calls this trail the "Oak Ridge Trail") continues straight ahead or for extra mileage, you can follow the White Tail Trail to the right for a 1.2-mile loop through an open field and skirting along the forest's edge. The park seems to have plenty of deer, look for signs of their presence (tracks, eating of bark). Stay on the Little Falls Trail/Oak Ridge Trail at this intersection by staying to the right until you come to the park road. Immediately before crossing the road is the Knapweed Trail (orange) named for a purple-blossomed wildflower that blooms late June through mid July. This 0.9-mile trail will take you back to the Pioneer Trail about 300 yards to the left of the parking lot where this hike started.

A shortcut at the intersection with the Knapweed Trail is to cross the road at the orange trail and connect with the Pioneer Trail (yellow). This is about 500 yards west of the starting point at the park entrance parking lot. Take the Pioneer Trail to the right and behind the parking lot. A short spur (the same one you took from the lot at the very beginning) leads back to your right into the parking lot.

NEARBY ACTIVITIES
The Wisconsin town of Hudson offers small river-town charm, shops, restaurants.

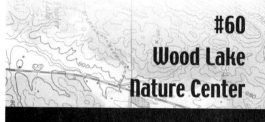

#60
Wood Lake
Nature Center

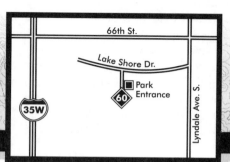

IN BRIEF

One block from one of the busiest shopping intersections in Richfield, flanked by freeways and houses…yet still one of the best marsh areas in Twin Cities. Lots of bird viewing opportunities and casual walking. Great close-ups of birds for aspiring photographers.

DIRECTIONS

From St. Paul/Minneapolis drive south on Interstate 35 West to 66th Street exit, go east to Lyndale Avenue and turn right (south). Drive 0.1 mile and turn left onto Lake Shore Drive at the sign to Wood Lake Nature Center. Park in the lot on the left.

DESCRIPTION

Whoever decided to put trails through and around marshy areas within the cities rather than drain them should be commended! These islands of nature surrounded by ribbons of concrete offer some of the best escapes from the everyday commotion of the "thriving metropolis" that otherwise consume such spaces. To understand and appreciate this concept better, spend some time at Wood Lake.

Here is an example of the marshlands so common to Minnesota—either in the form of shoreline along a secluded lake or as part of a pond in a glacially sculpted hardwood forest. Wood Lake represents an ecology common throughout

KEY AT-A-GLANCE INFORMATION

Length: 2.2 miles

Configuration: Figure eight loop with outer connecting loop

Difficulty: Very easy; flat and paved for the most part

Scenery: A vast marsh with several small ponds, tree lined to keep the eye from wandering beyond to the freeway

Exposure: Full sun except in wooded sections

Traffic: Popular throughout day, especially at lunch and right after work

Trail Surface: Paved or hard packed earth; solid wood-like surface on all floating docks

Hiking Time: 1–1¼ hours

Season: All seasons; best in summer

Access: No fees

Maps: Available at the visitor center

Facilities: Visitor center with rest rooms, interpretive displays, small picnic area, water

Special Comments: Plenty of parking in lot adjacent to visitor center

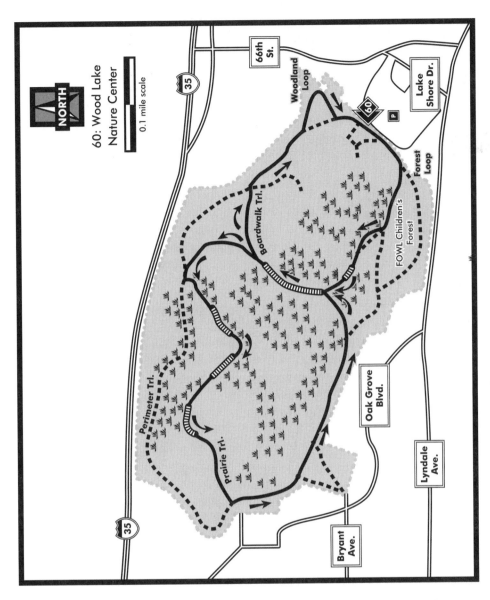

60: Wood Lake Nature Center

NORTH

0.1 mile scale

66th St.

Woodland Loop

Lake Shore Dr.

Forest Loop

Boardwalk Trl.

FOWL Children's Forest

Perimeter Trl.

Prairie Trl.

Oak Grove Blvd.

Lyndale Ave.

Bryant Ave.

this land of lakes. The trail system—laid out in a full-figured eight—takes hikers through a thoroughly representative sampling of Minnesota marshland.

The trail begins at the interpretive center and enables hikers to begin either a clockwise or counterclockwise progression along two loops that begin and end at the center. A short, 0.8-mile hike balloons out into the marsh and then

returns, while the larger 1.8-mile trail outlines the entire park. Combining the two in a large 2.2-mile figure eight allows hikers to enjoy all the trails in the park with but a few hundred yards of double-backs along the way.

Starting from the visitor center and going clockwise (south), you enter a corridor of stately cottonwoods, silver maples, and other lowland species that encircle the perimeter of Wood Park. At the first fork in the trail stay to the right, which also provides access to the observation docks near the center. (The left fork goes around the outside of the spindle-shaped Fowl Children's Forest—an interpretive area for visiting classrooms or classes put on by the center and around the outer perimeter of the park.) You'll encounter another fork 0.1 mile beyond the first one. Stay to the right to connect with the eastern section of the small trail loop. Follow this trail along the edge of the cattails and reeds.

If you follow the left side you can continue on along the outer perimeter of the park. The right fork cuts away from the Children's Forest about 0.1 mile beyond the fork and connects with the eastern section of the small trail loop. This is the trail you want for the first real glimpse of the marsh. Egrets and an occasional Great Blue Heron are frequent visitors here and you can usually find one or two standing as still as members of the Royal Guard. Blackbirds and swamp sparrows are among the residents in such marshy areas and Wood Lake is no different. They are perhaps the most common of the many species in this park. I've even seen one of the tern varieties flying overhead during the summer.

As you begin your way into the center of the marsh (via the center of the figure eight) you will be eye-to-eye with the profusion of cattails and reeds. Look carefully around the bases for bird activity, frogs, turtles, and even snakes. This area is alive with aquatic and terrestrial life. Sometimes the Canada geese, in the fall, will "take over" a section of the walkway. They will yield but not before a face-off. It's marshes like these that provide a bit of cover and rest for migrating flocks in the fall.

Resident mallards and coots are plentiful here, too. It's a great place for aspiring wildlife photographers to practice on most willing models. It's the proximity of the marshland to the viewer that is especially attractive about Wood Lake. Many of the parks and other areas provide access to and around marshes. Wood Lake enables you to actually walk through the marsh.

Continuing along the middle of the figure eight to the far side of the marsh, turn left and follow along the border of marshland and cottonwoods again. The right fork returns you to the visitor center—don't take it, there's still more to see!

The interior vegetation is made up of introduced species such as buckthorn, but the character of this border strip is that of an understory in a mixed forest stand. The tangle of understory is like that along the lowlands of the Mississippi a few miles away.

This strip of tall trees is also a good noise baffle for the ever-busy (and seemingly ever-under–construction) section of Interstate 35 West that connects the heart of Minneapolis with its southern suburbs across the river. Like the Mississippi, this interstate is handy connecting corridor to many more park units in the Twin Cities.

About another 0.1 mile from the middle fork the trail forks again. The left fork, the one you want to take, swings back through the marsh and connects with the Prairie Trail about 0.3 mile beyond the fork. It guides you through a drier part of the park adjacent to the marshes at the southern end. The other fork is the Perimeter Trail. This route skirts the extreme southern end of the park and outside edge of the prairie terrain. Both trails are about the same length.

The Prairie Trail eventually meets back up with the Perimeter Trail. Turn left and continue back along the last half of the big loop, once again encountering the big trees. Deer have been spotted here. There are numerous trails through the undergrowth—even though this borders on some homes. The trail leaves the marshes and openness, and flows through the dense forest of mature cottonwoods. Squirrels are common residents as are several varieties of woodpeckers including downy and hairy woodpeckers.

About 0.4 mile farther the trail forks again. Now you are back at the end of the Children's Forest near where you began. Take the left fork and again cross at the middle or waist of the figure eight. This is a short segment to re-hike but worth it since now you will approach the remaining section of the loop you have not yet hiked.

This is called the Boardwalk Trail. Turn right immediately upon reaching the other side of the marshes and head out to the observation dock that extends out into the marsh to near the edge of one of the half dozen ponds in the area. There is a trail through the woods that leads back to the main loop or you can double back along the dock trail and hang a hard right at that point. At about 0.15 mile you will meet up with the Woodland Loop that cuts into the deep woods for a 0.1-mile spur. The main trail continues on back to the visitors center.

NEARBY ACTIVITIES
Follow 66th Street east about 1 mile to Portland Avenue. Go about one block past Portland on 66th Street (east) and turn left into parking lot. This is another small park with a paved walking trail and floating walkway through marsh area. Great bird watching: egrets, grebes, coots, red-wing blackbirds, wood ducks, Canada geese.

Appendix—Information Sources

Anoka County Parks and Recreation
550 VBunker Lke Bulvd.
Andover, MN 55304
763-757-3920
www.anokacountyparks.com

Carver County Parks
10775 County Road 33
Young America, MN 55397
952-467-4200
www.co.carver.mn.us/publicworks/parks

City of Bloomington
2215 West Old Shakopee Road,
Bloomington, MN 55431
952-563-8877
www.ci.bloomington.mn.us

City of St. Paul
Division of Parks & Recreation
25d W. 4th St., Room 300
St., Paul. MN 55102
651-266-6400
www.stpaul.gov/parksrec

Dakota County Parks
8500 127th St. E.
Hastings, MN 55033
651-438-4660
651-438-4671 (24 hr. Info. Line)
www.co.dakota.mn.us/parks

Department of Natural Resources
State of Minnesota
500 Lafayette Road
St. Paul, MN 55155-4040

Info Center: 612-296-6157
1-888-MINNDNR
www.dnr.state.mn.us

Hennipen County Service Centers
612-348-8240 (General Information)

Hennepin Parks/Scott County
763-559-9000
www.hennepinparks.org

Minnesota Office of Tourism
800-657-3700
612-296-5029

Minneapolis Parks and Recreation Board
400 So. 4th St., Ste 200 Grain Exchange
Minneapolis, MN 55415-1400
612-661-4800
www.ci.minneapolis.mn.us/citywork/
other/park

Minnesota Valley National Wildlife Refuge
3815 E. 80th St.
Bloomington, MN 55425-1600
612-854-5900
http:midwest.fws.gov/minnesotavalley

Mississippi National River and Recreation Area
111 E. Kellogg Blvd., Ste. 105
St. Paul, MN 55101-1256
651-290-4160
www.nps.gov/miss

National Park Service
St. Croix National Scenic Riverway
651-430-1938
www.nps.gov/sacn

Ramsey County Parks and Recreation
2015 Van Dyke St.,
Maplewood, MN 55109
651-748-2500
www.co.ramsey.mn.us

Regional Parks; A Map and Guide
Metropolitan Council
Mears Park Center
230 E. fifth St.
St,. Paul, MN 55101-1626
651-602-1000
www.metrocouncil.org.

Suburban Hennepin Regional Park District
12615 Co. Rd 9
Plymouth, MN 55441
Trail Hotline: 763-559-6778

Washington County Parks
1515 Keats Ave. N.
Lake Elmo, MN 55042

651-430-8368
www.co.washington.mn.us/parks

U.S. Fish & Wildlife Service
1-800-344-WILD
www.usfws.gov

IN WISCONSIN

Association of Wisconsin Tourism Attractions (AWTA)
44 E. Mifflin Street, Ste. 900
Madison, WI 53703
1-800-372-2737
www.wistravel.com/AWTA

Wisconsin Department of Tourism
1-800-432-8747 / 1-800-372-2737
www.wistravel.com

Wisconsin Division of Natural Resources
Bureau of Parks and Recreation
P.O.Box 7921
Madison, WI 53707-7921
wiparks@dnr.state.wi.us
www.wiparks.net.
www.wistravel.com

Index

A

Abandon Falls Glen, 143
Afton Ski Area, 4
Afton State Park, 1–4
Alfalfa, winter-hardy strain, 200
Ann Lake, Sand Dunes State Forest, 5–7,
  186
Anoka, MN, 176
Archaeological digs
  arrowheads, 166
  Carver Park area, 199
  giant beaver remains, 148
Archery
  Mazomani Trail, 135
  Spring Lake Park Reserve, 193

B

Baker Near Wilderness Settlement, 10, 11
Bald eagles
  Kinnickinnic State Park, 92
  Minnesota NWR, 158
  Sherburne NWR, 185
Band shell, Lake Harriet, 31
Bandstand, Como Park, 98, 99
Barker Park Reserve, 8–11
Barn Bluff, 12–15
Bass Pond Trail, 16–19, 159
Bass-rearing ponds, 17
Basswood, 175, 210
Battle Creek, 20–22
Baylor Regional Park, 23–25
Beason Lake, 121
Bicycling. See also Mountain biking
  Battle Creek, 20, 21
  City Lakes Chain, 32
  Clearly Lake Regional Park, 34, 35
  Clifton E. French Regional Park, 39
  Fish Lake Regional Park, 64, 66
    Fort Snelling State Park, 69
    Lake Phalen area, 116
    Lake Rebecca Park, 118
    Mississippi Gorge Trail, 147, 148
    Old Cedar Avenue Trail, 158
    Pine Point Park Trail, 160
    Plymouth's bike/hike trail, 39
    Red Cedar Trail, 163, 166
    Rice Creek Chain of Lakes Park, 168,
      169
    Rice Creek West Regional Trail, 131
    Rum River Central, 173, 175
    Tamarack Trail, 197–198
    Vadnais Lake area, 189
"Big Woods" area
    Barker Park Reserve, 10
    Elm Creek Park Reserve, 61
    Lake Maria State Park, 103
    Lake Rebecca Park, 117
    overview, xx
    Sherburne NWR, 184
Big Woods Dairy, 155
Big Woods Trail, 152–155
Bird watching
    Barker Park Reserve, 10
    Bass Pond Trail/Long Meadow Lake, 16,
      17, 19
    Battle Creek, 22
    City Lakes Chain, 31–32
    Como Lake, 99
    Coon Rapids Dam, 42
    Crow-Hassen State Park, 53–54
    Eastman Nature Trail, 57, 58
    Frontenac State Park area, 72
    Holland/Jensen Lakes Loop, 127, 128
    Hyland Lakes Park Reserve, 80
    Kinnickinnic State Park, 92, 93
    Lake Rebecca Park, 119

Lawrence Trail, 122
list of hikes for, xvii
Mazomani Trail, 136, 137
Miesville Ravine Park, 139, 140
Murphy-Hanrehan Park, 151
Nerstrand Woods State Park, 155
Old Cedar Avenue Trail, 156, 157,
    158–159
Rice Creek Chain of Lakes Park, 169
Rice Lake State Park, 170, 171
Rum River Central, 173
Rum River North, 179
Sand Dunes State Forest, 7
Sherburne NWR, 183, 184, 185, 186
Tamarack Nature Center, 196
Tamarack Trail, 199, 200
Thompson Trail, 202
Wild River, 205
William O'Brien State Park, 211
Willow River, WI, 215
Wood Lake Nature Center, 216, 218,
    219
Black Dog Preserve, 159
Black Dog Trail, 69
Blanding's turtle, 103, 105
Boardwalks
Eastman Nature Trail, 57, 58
Lawrence Trail, 123
Boating. See also Canoeing; specific hikes
    "key at-a-glance information" facilities list
    Bryant Lake Figure Eight, 28
    Coon Rapids Dam, 42
    Rice Lake State Park, 170, 172
Bob Dunn Recreation Area, 5, 7
Botanical conservatory, Como Park, 97, 99
"Bottomless Pit", 84
Bryant Lake Figure Eight, 26–28
Burkhardt, Christian, 214
Business hiker, xxiii

C

Calhoun Beach Hotel, 31
Camping. See also specific hikes "key at-a-
    glance information" facilities list
    Rice Lake State Park, 172
    Wild River, 207
Cannon River, 94, 181
Canoeing
    Cannon River, 140

City Lakes chain, 31
Holland/Jensen Lakes Loop, 127
Interstate Park, 84, 85
Lake Maria State Park, 105, 106
Rice Creek Chain of Lakes Park, 169
Rice Lake State Park, 170
Rum River Central, 174, 175, 176
Wild River, 204, 207
Carver, Jonathan, 12
Carver Park Reserve, 196, 197, 199
Carver Rapids Loop, 136, 137
Cedar Lake, 30, 31, 113
Cenaiko Trout Lake, 42
Centerville Lake, 168, 169
Children
    hikes for, xvi–xvii
    hiking with, xxiii
Chippewa Native Americans, 213
Chippewa River, 166
Chippewa River State Trail, 166
City Lakes Chain (Lakes Harriet, Calhoun,
    Isles), 29–32
Clearly Lake Regional Park, 33–36, 151
Clifton E. French Regional Park, 37–39, 66
Clothing/shoes for hiking, xxii–xxiii
Como Park, 97–99
Como Park Zoo, 97, 99
Contact information, 220–221
Coon Rapids Dam, 40–42
Cottage Grove Ravine Regional Park,
    43–46
Cottonwood trees
    Crosby Farm Park, 49
    Fort Snelling State Park, 67, 68
    Frontenac State Park area, 72
    Long Lake, 131
Crosby, Thomas and Emma, 47–48
Crosby Farm Park, 47–50, 69, 148
Crosby Lake, 198, 199
Cross-country skiing. See Skiing
Crow-Hassen State Park, 51–54
Crow River, 53, 118
Cryptosporidium, xxii
Cycling. See Bicycling

D

Dairy industry, 200
Dakota Native Americans, 69, 71, 133–134
Dalles of the St. Croix River, 82, 84, 86, 87

Devil's Punch Bowl, 165
Driftless Area, 165
Ducks Unlimited, 135
Dunnville National Wildlife Refuge, 166
Dwarf trout lily, 152, 155

E

Eagle Lake, 24, 25
Eagle Point Lake, 100–102
Eastern red cedars, 94–95
Eastman Nature Center, 55, 57, 61, 63
Eastman Nature Trail, 55–59
Ecological regions, xx
Ecotone, 182
Education centers. *See* Interpretive trails;
    Nature centers
Ehmiller Farmstead, 134, 135
Elm Creek Park Reserve
    description, 60–63
    Eastman Nature Trail, 55–59
    proximity to other trails, 42, 66, 131,
        175–176
Etiquette on trails, xxi

F

Fall foliage
    Lake Byllesby Regional Park, 96
    list of hikes for, xvii
    Mazomani Trail, 135
Faribault, Jean Baptiste, 134
Fire tower, Sand Dunes State Forest, 6–7
First-aid kit, xxii
Fish Lake Regional Park, 64–66
Fishing
    Bass Pond Trail/Long Meadow Lake, 17
    Bryant Lake Figure Eight, 28
    Clifton E. French Regional Park,
        37, 39
    Coon Rapids Dam, 42
    Fish Lake Regional Park, 66
    Hay Creek, 77
    Kinnickinnic River, 91, 93
    Lake Como, 98
    Medicine Lake, 39
    Minnehaha Creek/Falls, 144
    Singing Hills Trail, 181
Flora, list of hikes for, xvii
Ford Bridge, 144, 145, 148
Fort Snelling State Park, 47-48, 50, 67–69

Fox Native Americans, 71
Frontenac Golf Course, 73
Frontenac State Park, 15, 70–73

G

Gateway Trail, 116
Geographic features, list of hikes for, xvii
Geology
    Barn Bluff, 13
    Carver Park area, 199
    Clifton E. French Regional Park, 38
    Frontenac State Park, 70–71
    Lake Rebecca Park, 117
    Mississippi Gorge Trail, 147
    Nerstrand Woods State Park, 154
    Old Cedar Avenue Trail, 159
    Red Cedar River, 165
    Rice Lake State Park, 171, 172
    Sakatah State Park, 182
    Twin Cities area, xx
Giardia, xxii
Gilboa, Mt., 81
Glacial Lake Agassiz, 122, 159
Glacial River Warren, 70, 122, 159
Glaciers
    Barn Bluff, 13
    Clearly Lake Regional Park, 33
    Clifton E. French Regional Park, 38
    Hyland Lakes Park Reserve, 80
    Interstate Park, MN, 82, 84
    Interstate Park, WI, 86–88
    Lake Calhoun, 31
    lake formation by, 31
    Lake Maria State Park, 103–104
    Lawrence Trail, 122
    Mazomani Trail, 136
    Minnesota lakes and, 31
    Murphy-Hanrehan Park Reserve,
        150–151
    Nerstrand Woods State Park, 154
    Old Cedar Avenue Trail, 159
    Rice Lake State Park, 171
    Sakatah State Park, 182
    St. Croix Valley, 208
    Thompson Trail, 202
Golf
    Como Park, 97
    Frontenac Golf Course, 73
    Lake Phalen area, 114, 116

Rice Creek Chain of Lakes Park, 168, 169
Grand Rounds Trail, 110
Grass Lake, 188, 189
Great Northern Railroad, 200
"Green tree reservoir", 18
Grimm Farm, 200

H

Hamm's Memorial Waterfall, 98
Handicapped accessibility. *See* Wheelchairs
Hardwoods region, xx
Hay Creek, 15
Hay Creek, West Trail, 74–77
Hay Creek Management Unit, 74–75
Hennepin, Louis (Father), 71
Hennepin-Lake area, 32
Hennepin Regional Park District, 117–118
Hiawatha statue, 141
Hidden Falls
  on Mississippi River, 50, 148
  Nerstrand Woods State Park, 154, 155
Hikes
  with children, xvi, xxiii
  by difficulty, xvi-xvii
  locations, viii-ix
  by mileage, xv-xvi
  multi-use trail list, xvi
  recommendations, xv-xvii
Hill, James J., 200
Historical sites
  Crosby Farm Park, 47-48
  Fort Snelling State Park, 67–69
  Frontenac State Park, 71–72, 73
  Lawrence Trail, 122
  list of hikes for, xvii
  Long Lake, 129, 130–131, 132
  Mazomani Trail, 133–135, 136
  Rice Lake State Park, 170, 172
  Willow River, WI, 213–214
Holland/Jensen Lakes Loop, 124–128
Hopewellian culture, 71
Horse trails
  Barker Park Reserve, 9, 10–11
  Crow-Hasssen State Park, 51, 52
  Elm Creek Park Reserve, 62, 63
  Hay Creek Management Unit, 74, 75–76
  Holland/Jensen Lakes Loop, 127, 128

Lake Maria State Park, 105
Lawrence Trail, 120, 121
Murphy-Hanrehan Park Reserve, 149
Pine Point Park Trail, 160
Rum River Central, 173, 175
Wild River, 205
Hudson, WI, 214, 215
Hunting
  Hay Creek Management Unit, 75
  Holland/Jensen Lakes Loop, 128
  Mazomani Trail, 135
Hyland Lakes Park Reserve, 78–81

I

Ice house remnants, 131
Ice Palisades, 165
Indian Mounds Park, 22
Information sources, 220–221
Inline skating
  City Lakes Chain, 32
  Pine Point Park Trail, 160
Interpretive trails
  Eastman Nature Trail, 55–59, 63
  Frontenac State Park, 72, 73
  Long Lake, 130–131
  Tamarack Nature Center, 196
  Wood Lake Nature Center, 218
Interstate Park, MN, 82–85, 211
Interstate Park, WI, 86–90
Ironwood trees, 106, 119

J

Jabs Farm, 134, 135, 136
Jack pine, 7
Jensen/Holland Lakes Loop, Lebanon Hills Regional Park, 124–128
John Steven's house, 144

K

"Kames", 150, 203
Kayaking
  Cannon River, 140
  Interstate Park, 84
Keller Golf Course, 114–115, 116
Keller Lake, 116
Keller Park/Picnic Area, 116
"Kettles", 150, 151, 203
Kinnickinnic River, 91–92, 93
Kinnickinnic State Park, 91–93

L

Lake Agassiz, 122, 159
Lake Bjorkland, 105
Lake Byllesby Regional Park, 94–96
Lake Calhoun, 29, 30, 31, 113
Lake Como, 97–99
Lake Elmo Park Reserve, 100–102
Lake Harriet, 29–31, 32, 113
Lake Itasca, 146–147
Lake Katrina, 8, 9
Lake Louise, 161, 162
Lake Maria State Park, 103–106
Lake Minnewashta Regional Park, 107–109
Lake Nokomis, 29, 110–113
Lake O' the Dalles, 86, 89–90
Lake of the Isles, 29, 30, 31–32, 113
Lake Phalen, 114–116
Lake Rebecca Park, 54, 117–119
Lake Sarah Park, 119
Lake Superior, 87
Landscaping for wildlife, 56
Lava, 87
Lawrence Trail, Minnesota Valley, 120–123
Lebanon Hills Regional Park, 124–128
Linden, 175, 210
Little Bluestem Pool, 185
Lock and Dam Number One, 144, 148
Logging, 206–207, 214
Long, Stephen H., 13
Long Lake, 129–132
Long Meadow Lake
    Bass Pond Trail, 16–19
    Old Cedar Avenue Trail, 156–159
Longfellow, 141
Loon Lake, 161
Louisville Swamp, 120, 123, 133, 134–135, 136–137
Lowry Nature Center, 196, 197–200
Luce Line Trail Corridor, 11

M

Mall of America, 16, 19
Maps
    legend, vii
    topo maps, xx–xxi
Marine-On-St. Croix, 162
Marsh Trail, Lake Minnewashta Regional Park, 107–109
Mazomani (Chief), 133

Mazomani Trail, 133–137
Medicine Lake, 37, 38, 39
Mesic oak savanna, 148
Miesville Ravine Park, 15, 96, 138–140
Mille Lacs Lake, 174
Minnehaha Creek, 110, 113, 141–144
Minnehaha Falls, 29, 50, 110, 113, 141–144
Minnehaha statue, 141
Minnehaha Trail, 69
Minnesota Arboretum, 109
Minnesota River. See also Minnesota Valley
    Crosby Farm Park, 47, 48
    Fort Snelling State Park, 67, 68
    Lawrence Trail, 120, 121
Minnesota Valley
    Lawrence Trail, 120–123
    Louisville Swamp, 120, 123, 133, 134–135, 136–137
Mazomani Trail, 133–137
Minnesota Valley National Wildlife
    Refuge, 16–19, 134, 156.
        See also specific hikes
Minnesota Zoo, 128
Mississippi Gorge Trail, 29, 145–148
Mississippi National River and Recreation
    Area (MNRRA), 145–146
Mississippi River
    Barn Bluff, 12
    Coon Rapids Dam, 40, 41, 42
    Crosby Farm Park, 47–48, 49
    Fort Snelling State Park, 67, 68, 69
    Frontenac State Park, 70, 71–72, 73
    Minnehaha Creek and, 142, 144
    Richard J. Dorer Memorial Hardwood
    State Forest, 75
    Rum River and, 174
    Spring Lake Park Reserve and, 190, 191, 192
    Thompson Trail and, 203
Mountain biking
    Afton State Park, 4
    Hyland Park, 81
Murphy-Hanrehan Park Reserve, 149, 150, 151
Mt. Gilboa, 81
Mud Lake, 63
Munger State Trail, 160, 161, 162
Murphy-Hanrehan Park, 34–35, 36, 149–151

N

National Ice Age Reserve, 86
Native Americans
  Chippewa, 213
  Dakota, 69, 71, 133–134
  Fox, 71
  Frontenac State Park and, 73
  Minnehaha Creek/Falls and, 143
  Sioux, 182, 213
  Wahpekita, 180
Nature centers
  Crosby Farm Park, 47
  Eastman Nature Center, 55, 57, 61, 63
  Lowry Nature Center, 196, 197–200
  Richardson Nature Center, 78–79, 81
  Tamarack Nature Center, 194–196
  Wood Lake Nature Center, 216–219
Nerstrand Woods State Park, 96, 152–155
Nevers Dam site, 206–207
New Brighton, MN, 130–131
Nine Mile Creek, 28
North Hennepin Regional Trail, 42
Northern Conifers region, xx

O

Oak savannas
  overview, xx
  as rare plant community, 148
  Rum River Central, 173–174
  Sherburne NWR, 184
O'Brien Lake, 125, 126
Old Cedar Avenue Trail, 156–159
Old Soldiers Home bridge, 144
Omni Theatre, Minnesota Zoo, 128

P

Perrant, "Pig's Eye", 48
Pet trails
  Clifton E. French Park, 38–39
  Hyland Lakes Park Reserve, 78
Petroglyphs, 166
Phalen Golf Course, 116
Picnic areas. See also specific hikes "key at-a-
  glance information" facilities list
  Crosby Farm Park, 49, 50
  Crow-Hassen State Park, 53
  Holland/Jensen Lakes Loop, 126
  Lake Maria State Park, 105
  Lake Phalen area, 114, 115, 116

Long Lake, 131
  Minnehaha Creek/Falls, 144
  Red Cedar Trail, 166
  Rice Lake State Park, 170
  Rum River North, 178, 179
  Singing Hills Trail, 181
  Spring Lake Park Reserve, 192
  Tamarack Trail, 199
  Wild River, 206, 207
"Pig's Eye" Perrant, 48
Pike, Zebulon, 69
Pike Island, 47–48, 50, 67
Pine Point Park Trail, 160–162
Pinelands region, xx
Plymouth's bike/hike trail, 39
Point Douglas Park, 46
Point No Point, 72, 109
Poison ivy, xxii
Potholes
  Interstate Park, 82, 84, 87–88
  Lake Maria State Park, 103
Prairie Creek, 153, 154
Prairie Lake, 53
Prairie restoration
  Crow-Hassen State Park, 51, 53
  Hylands Lakes Park Reserve, 81
  Kinnickinnic State Park, 91, 92, 93
  Tamarack Nature Center, 194
Prairies
  Hyland Lakes Park Reserve, 78, 79, 81
  overview, xx
Prairie's Edge Trail, 183–186
Prescott, WI, 46, 91, 92, 93
Prickly ash, xxii, 56, 140
Putnam Lake, 105

Q

Quarry sites
  Frontenac State Park, 72
  Red Cedar Trail, 166

R

Rails-to-trails paths, 165, 180, 181
Rattail Lake, 119
Red Cedar Junction Line, 165
Red Cedar River, 163, 164, 165, 166
Red Cedar Trail, 163–166
Red Wing, MN, 12, 14, 15, 77
Renaissance Fair, 137

Reshanau Lake, 169
Rice Creek Chain of Lakes Park, 1
   67–169
Rice Creek West Regional Trail, 131
Rice Lake State Park, 96, 170–172
Richard J. Dorer Memorial Hardwood
   State Forest, 74–75
Richardson Nature Center, 78–79, 81
River Warren, 70, 122, 159
Riverboat tours, St. Croix River, xiii, 85
Rose Garden, Lake Harriet, 32
Rum River Central, 173–176
Rum River North, 177–179
Rush Creek, 59
Russell A. Sorenson Landing, 159

S

Sakatah Lake State Park, 180–182
Sand Dunes State Forest, 5–7, 186
Sand plains, xx
Schaar's Bluff Trail, 190–193
Schoolhouse, Minnesota's oldest, 85
Sherburne NWR, 5, 183–186
Shoes/clothing for hiking, xxii–xxiii
Showy lady slipper, 62
Silver Lake, 106
Singing Hills Trail, 96, 180–181, 182
Sioux Native Americans, 182, 213
Skiing
   Afton Ski Area, 4
   Battle Creek, 21
   Clearly Lake Regional Park, 34, 36
   Hay Creek Management Unit, 75
   Holland/Jensen Lakes Loop, 127, 128
   Marsh Trail, 108
   Mazomani Trail, 135
   Murphy-Hanrehan Park Reserve, 149,
      151
   Rice Lake State Park, 172
   Tamarack Nature Center, 196
   William O'Brien State Park, 210
Snail Lake, 187–189, 196
Snowmobiling
   Sand Dunes State Forest, 7
   Tamarack Trail, 199
Snowshoeing
   Afton Ski Area, 4
   Elm Creek Park Reserve, 61
"Song of Hiawatha", 141

Spring Lake Park Reserve, 190–193
St. Croix Moraines, xx
St. Croix River
   Afton State Park, 2, 3
   Interstate Park, 82–84, 85, 86–87, 88, 89
   Kinnickinnic River and, 91, 92, 93
   Mississippi River confluence, 43, 45, 190
   Wild River State Park, 204, 205, 206, 207
   William O'Brien State Park and, 208, 211
State Trail Corridor, 137
Steven's, John,, 144
Stillwater, MN, 162
Stinging nettle, xxii
Strait, Samuel B., homestead, 122
Strollers on trails, 194–195
Sunrise River, 206, 207
Swales, 28
Swimming
   Afton State Park, 3–4
   Clearly Lake Regional Park, 35, 36
   Clifton E. French Regional Park, 37
   Lake Harriet, 32
   Lake Nokomis, 113
   Lake Phalen, 114, 116
   Red Cedar Trail, 166

T

Tamarack Nature Center, 194–196
Tamarack Trail, Lowry Nature Center,
   197–200
Tamarack trees, 194, 196, 198–199
Taylor's Falls, MN, 85
Taylor's Landing, 82
Teal Pool, 184, 185
Tennis
   Baylor Regional Park, 25
   City Lakes Chain, 32
Thomas Beach, Lake Calhoun, 31
Thompson County Park, 201–203
Thompson Lake, 201, 202
Thompson Trail, 201–203
Thoreau, Henry David, 12–13
Tree-finder/identifier, 206
Trout lily, dwarf, 152, 155
Trout rivers/streams
   Hay Creek, 77
   Kinnickinnic River, 91, 93
   Willow River, 214
Trumpeter Swan Refuge, 10

Trumpeter swans, 10, 53, 103
Turkeys, 61, 93

U

Uncas Dunes Scientific and Nature Area, 5
U.S. Geological Survey topographic maps,
 xx–xxi

V

Vadnais Lake, 187, 189, 196
Vita-Course, Lake Nokomis, 112
Volleyball
 Baylor Regional Park, 25
 near Lake Calhoun, 31

W

Wahapetonwan tribe, 133–134
Wahpekita Native Americans, 180
Water for hiking, xxi–xxii
Weather overview, xix–xx
Welch Village, 140
Wetland drainage, 135
Wheat industry, 214
Wheelchairs
 Rice Creek Chain of Lakes Park, 167,
  168
 Tamarack Nature Center, 194–195
White pines, 7
Wild rice lakes, 213
Wild River, 204–207
Wildflowers
 Mazomani Trail, 135
 Miesville Ravine Park, 139
 Minnehaha Creek/Falls, 143
 Nerstrand Woods State Park, 152, 155
 Tamarack Nature Center, 194

Tamarack Trail, 199
 William O'Brien State Park, 211
Wildlife. *See also* Bird watching
 Carver Park area, 199
 Eastman Nature Trail, 58
 Elm Creek Park Reserve, 61
 Fort Snelling State Park, 69
 Hyland Lakes Park Reserve, 81
 Lake Elmo Park Reserve, 102
 Lake Maria State Park, 103, 105, 106
 Mazomani Trail, 137
 Miesville Ravine Park, 139
 Murphy-Hanrehan Park, 151
 Old Cedar Avenue Trail, 157–158
 Pine Point Park Trail, 162
 Sherburne NWR, 184, 185
 Tamarack Nature Center, 194
Willow River, WI, 215
Wood Lake Nature Center, 218, 219
Willard Munger State Trail, 160, 161, 162
William O'Brien State Park, 162, 207,
 208–211
William Scott Grave Site, 213, 214
Willow Falls, 212, 214–215
Willow River, WI, 212–215
Wood Lake Nature Center, 216–219
Work Projects Administration (WPA), 18

Z

Zoos
 Como Park Zoo, 97, 99
 Minnesota Zoo, 128
Zumbro River, 171

About the Author

Born in California, Tom Watson moved to the Twin Cities from Missouri at age seven. He remained in Minnesota until graduating from the College of Forestry of the University of Minnesota with B.S. in Forest Resource Management/Recreation. Then, in the mid-1980s, Tom moved to Kodiak Alaska, where he spent 15 years operating a sea kayak touring business and began working as a freelance writer and photographer. Published in several national magazines and an active member of the Outdoor Writers Association of America, Tom has won several awards for his articles. Besides hiking, his hobbies include photography, music, community theatre, gardening, bird-watching, paddling, and camping.